LEAN AND GREEN COOKBOOK FOR BEGINNERS 2022

1200 Days Fueling Hacks & Lean and Green Recipes to Burn Fat, Lose Weight, and Achieve a Healthy Lifestyle By Harnessing the Power of 5&1 and 4&2&1 Meal Plan

TABLE OF CONTENTS

INTRODUCTION..4

CHAPTER 1. WHAT IS A LEAN AND GREEN DIET?.............5

What Do You Eat on a Lean and Green Diet? 5
What is Fueling?.. 6
Foods to Avoid 6
How Often Do You Eat on a Lean and Green Diet?........... 6
How Does Lean and Green Diet Work for Weight Loss?.... 7

CHAPTER 2. WHAT ARE THE BENEFITS OF THE LEAN AND GREEN DIET? 8

Easy to Follow 8
May Improve Blood Pressure 9
It Offers Continuous Support 9
Achieves Fast Weight Loss 9
It Removes Guesswork 9

CHAPTER 3. BREAKFAST RECIPES 10

1. Oatmeal Yogurt... 10
2. Muesli Smoothie Bowl 10
3. Fried Egg with Bacon 11
4. Grain Bread and Avocado 11
5. Porridge with Walnuts 12
6. Mango Granola... 12
7. Blueberry & Cashew Waffles............................. 13
8. Eggless Scramble 13
9. Broccoli Waffles 14
10. Strawberry Yogurt Treats 14
11. Apple Oatmeal 15
12. Kale Scramble 15
13. Cheesy Flax and Hemp Seeds Muffins 16
14. Cheddar Broccoli Bread................................. 16
15. Pomegranate, Nuts and Chia 17
16. Bacon and Brussels Sprout Breakfast 17
17. Blueberry Moss Pancakes 18
18. Banana Cashew Toast 18
19. Eggs and Avocado Toast 19
20. Cheesy Spinach Waffles 19
21. Swiss Chard and Spinach with Egg 20
22. Avocado Chicken Salad 20
23. Yogurt with Granola and Persimmon 21
24. Vegan-Friendly Banana Bread 21

CHAPTER 4. LUNCH RECIPES 22

25. Salmon Burgers... 22
26. Stuffed Mushrooms....................................... 22
27. Mini Mac in a Bowl 23
28. Zucchini Frittata.. 23
29. Chicken Omelet 24
30. Chicken Pesto Pasta 24
31. Crab Cakes 25
32. Cayenne Rib Eye Steak 25
33. Pasta with Avocado and Cream......................... 26

34. Spaghetti Squash with Cheese and Pesto 26
35. Eggs in Pepper Rings.................................... 27
36. Fish Lettuce Tacos....................................... 27
37. Meatball Lasagna.. 28
38. Lettuce Salad with Beef Strips.......................... 28
39. Mozzarella, Tomatoes and Pesto Chicken 29
40. Cheesy Jalapeños.. 29
41. Avocados Stuffed with Salmon......................... 30
42. Chicken Gordon Bleu 30
43. Smoked Salmon with Avocado Oil...................... 31
44. Lemon Parmesan Salmon 31
45. Tasty Pancakes... 32
46. Tuna Cobbler... 32
47. Bacon Frittatawith Asparagus 33
48. Spaghetti Squash Casserole 33

CHAPTER 5. SNACK RECIPES 34

49. Cauliflower Pizza with Chicken & Tzatziki 34
50. 2-Ingredient Peanut Butter Energy Bites 34
51. Thin Mint Cookies.. 35
52. Red Velvet Whoopie Pies 35
53. Mint Chocolate Cheesecake Muffins 36
54. Neapolitan Froyo Popsicles............................. 36
55. Pizza, Spaghetti and Marinara Sauce................... 37
56. Cranberry Sweet Potato Muffins 37
57. Mini Peanut Butter Cups 38
58. Skinny Chicken Queso................................... 38
59. Personal Biscuit Pizza 39
60. Mini Cranberry Orange Spiced Cheesecake........... 39
61. Caprese Pizza Bites 40
62. Silky Peanut Butter Cookies 40
63. Smash Potato Grilled Cheese 41
64. Buffalo Cauliflower Wings 41
65. Cheddar & Chive Savory Smashed Potato Waffles 42
66. Very Veggie Dip 42
67. Pinto's & Cheese Fueling Hack 43
68. Personal Portobello Mushroom Pizzas 43
69. Grilled Mahi with Jicama Slaw.......................... 44
70. Taco Stuffed Portobellos 44
71. Mini Pepper Nachos 45
72. Curried Chicken Salad Wraps 45
73. Cilantro Lime Fish 46
74. West Indies Shrimp....................................... 46

CHAPTER 6. DINNER RECIPES 47

75. Air Fryer Asparagus...................................... 47
76. Avocado Fries.. 47
77. Cheesy Zucchini 48
78. Veggie Crusty Pizza 48
79. Tarragon Cauliflower..................................... 49
80. Winter Salad 49
81. Energizing Mocha Smoothie 50
82. Flavored Sandwich Filling 50
83. Angelic Pasta... 51

84. FREE TOFU 51
85. UNFORGETTABLE MASHED POTATOES 52
86. TURKEY MEATBALLS WITH HERBS 52
87. ZUCCHINI SALMON SALAD 53
88. PAN FRIED SALMON 53
89. MOUSSAKA WITH PAPRIKA 54
90. TUNA SALAD 54
91. CUCUMBER YOGURT 55
92. LIME TARRAGON DRESSING 55
93. FANTASTIC SALMON SALAD 56
94. JUICY FRIED SALMON 56
95. SALMON WITH PINEAPPLE 57
96. GREEK FISH 57
97. VEGGIES AND FISH BAKE 58
98. BEEF WITH MUSHROOMS 58

CHAPTER 7. SMOOTHIE RECIPES 59

99. GREEN COLADA SMOOTHIE 59
100. GREEN APPLE SMOOTHIE 59
101. REFRESHING LIME SMOOTHIE 60
102. BROCCOLI GREEN SMOOTHIE 60
103. APPLE SPINACH CUCUMBER SMOOTHIE 61
104. GREEN MANGO SMOOTHIE 61
105. SWEET GREEN SMOOTHIE 62
106. SUPER HEALTHY GREEN SMOOTHIE 62
107. SPINACH SMOOTHIE 63
108. SPINACH PEACH BANANA SMOOTHIE 63
109. SPINACH COCONUT SMOOTHIE 64
110. SALTY GREEN SMOOTHIE 64
111. WATERMELON STRAWBERRY SMOOTHIE 65
112. AVOCADO MANGO SMOOTHIE 65
113. CHIA SEED SMOOTHIE 66
114. MATCHA AVOCADO SMOOTHIE 66
115. HEALTHY GREEN SMOOTHIE 67
116. MANGO SMOOTHIE 67
117. WATERMELON KALE SMOOTHIE 68
118. MIX BERRY WATERMELON SMOOTHIE 68
119. PLUM AND AVOCADO SMOOTHIE 68
120. CREAMY RASPBERRY POMEGRANATE SMOOTHIE 69
121. LEAN AND GREEN SMOOTHIE 1 69
122. PUMPKIN SMOOTHIE 69

CHAPTER 8. FISH AND SEAFOOD RECIPES 70

123. DILL RELISH ON WHITE SEA BASS 70
124. SUMMER SHRIMP PRIMAVERA 70
125. GRILLED SALMON WITH CUCUMBER DILL SAUCE 71
126. SHRIMP AND ENDIVES 72
127. BASIL 'N LIME-CHILI CLAMS 72
128. BAKED FISH FILLETS 73
129. GRILLED SPLIT LOBSTER 73
130. FISH BONE BROTH 74
131. SALMON CAKES 74
132. LEMON AIOLI AND SWORDFISH PANINI 75
133. SALMON WITH MUSTARD 75
134. DIJON MUSTARD AND LIME MARINATED SHRIMP 76
135. BREADED AND SPICED HALIBUT 76
136. CILANTRO SHRIMP 77
137. GARLICKY CLAMS 77
138. LEMON SWORDFISH 78
139. BAKED SCALLOPS WITH GARLIC AIOLI 78
140. TILAPIA TACOS 79
141. SALMON WITH VEGGIES 79
142. LEMON, BUTTERED SHRIMP PANINI 80
143. BAKED COD CRUSTED WITH HERBS 80
144. CRAZY SAGANAKI SHRIMP 81

CHAPTER 9. POULTRY RECIPES 82

145. POPPIN' POP CORN CHICKEN 82
146. CHICKEN BREAST WITH ASPARAGUS 82
147. CHICKEN WITH BELL PEPPERS 83
148. VINEGAR CHICKEN 83
149. CHICKEN WITH ZOODLES 84
150. CHICKEN AND CAULIFLOWER 84
151. CHICKEN AND BOK CHOY 85
152. CHICKEN & STRAWBERRY LETTUCE WRAPS 85
153. ORANGE CHICKEN 86
154. CHICKEN STUFFED AVOCADO 86
155. CHICKEN & VEGGIES STIR FRY 87
156. CHICKEN & BROCCOLI BAKE 87
157. CHEESY CHICKEN & SPINACH 88
158. CHICKEN WITH MUSHROOMS 88
159. WHOLE CHICKEN ROAST 89
160. BASIL DUCK FILLET 89
161. CHICKEN WITH BROCCOLI & MUSHROOMS 90
162. CHICKEN & ASPARAGUS FRITTATA 90
163. CHICKEN & ZUCCHINI MUFFINS 91
164. CHICKEN & BELL PEPPER MUFFINS 91
165. CHICKEN STROGANOFF 92

CHAPTER 10. VEGAN & VEGETARIAN RECIPES 93

166. QUINOA PORRIDGE 93
167. POTATO HASH WITH CILANTRO-LIME CREAM 93
168. MILLET PORRIDGE 94
169. CRUNCHY QUINOA MEAL 94
170. BANANA BARLEY PORRIDGE 95
171. PUMPKIN SPICE QUINOA 95
172. BAKED CHEESY EGGPLANT WITH MARINARA 96
173. BABY CORN IN CHILI-TURMERIC SPICE 96
174. JACKFRUIT VEGETABLE FRY 97
175. ZUCCHINI NOODLES WITH CREAMY AVOCADO PESTO 97
176. CELERIAC STUFFED AVOCADO 98
177. BAKED POTATO TOPPED WITH CREAM CHEESE AND OLIVES 98
178. PEANUT SAUCE, GREEN VEGETABLES AND TEMPEH 99
179. SPICY WAFFLE WITH JALAPENO 99
180. GREEN PEA GUACAMOLE 100
181. HEMP SEED PORRIDGE 100
182. COCONUT PANCAKES 101
183. VEGGIE FRITTERS 101
184. ASPARAGUS WITH GARLIC 102
185. BLACK BEANS AND SWEET POTATO TACOS 102
186. BAKED PORTOBELLO, PASTA, AND CHEESE 103

CHAPTER 11. PORK RECIPES 104

187. PORK RIND NACHOS 104

188. AIR FRYER WHOLE WHEAT CRUSTED PORK CHOPS......... 104
189. PORK CHOP WITH BRUSSELS SPROUT 105
190. PORK DUMPLINGS WITH SAUCE 105
191. MOZZARELLA PORK BELLY CHEESE 106
192. PANKO CRUSTED PORK CHOPS 107
193. APPLE STUFFY PORK CHOP 107
194. AIR FRYER PORK CHOP & BROCCOLI............................ 108
195. JUICY PORK CHOPS 108
196. SUPER EASY PORK CHOPS.. 109
197. NO BREAD PORK BELLY... 109
198. CREAMY PORK BELLY ROLLS..................................... 110
199. SEASONED BLEU PORK BELLY 110
200. MUSTARD GLAZED AIR FRYER PORK TENDERLOIN 111
201. RUSTIC PORK RIBS 111
202. PORK TENDERLOIN 112
203. QUICK PORK BELLY 112
204. CRISPY PORK CUTLETS 113
205. SOUTHERN STYLE PORK CHOPS................................ 113
206. ROASTED PEPPER PORK PROSCIUTTO.......................... 114
207. EASY COOK PORK 114

CHAPTER 12. APPETIZER RECIPES 115

208. CAULIFLOWER RICE 115
209. BELL-PEPPER WRAPPED IN TORTILLA.......................... 115
210. ZUCCHINI OMELET 116
211. CHEESY CAULIFLOWER FRITTERS 116
212. ZUCCHINI PARMESAN CHIPS 117
213. JALAPENO CHEESE BALLS....................................... 117
214. CRISPY ROASTED BROCCOLI 118
215. COCONUT BATTERED CAULIFLOWER BITES.................... 118
216. CRISPY JALAPENO COINS 119
217. BUFFALO CAULIFLOWER 119
218. CARROT CAKE OATMEAL 120
219. SPICED SORGHUM AND BERRIES 120
220. PLANT-POWERED PANCAKES 121
221. SWEET CASHEW CHEESE SPREAD 121
222. CRISPY CAULIFLOWERS... 122
223. PESTO ZUCCHINI NOODLES 122
224. HERBED WILD RICE 123
225. BEEF WITH BROCCOLI OR CAULIFLOWER RICE 123
226. BARLEY RISOTTO 124
227. RISOTTO WITH GREEN BEANS AND SWEET POTATOES 124
228. MAPLE LEMON TEMPEH CUBES 125
229. QUINOA WITH VEGETABLES 125

CHAPTER 13. SOUPS AND SALADS 126

230. WASABI TUNA ASIAN SALAD.................................... 126
231. CALIFORNIA SOUP... 126
232. CHEESY CAULIFLOWER SOUP................................... 127
233. EGG DROP SOUP 127
234. CAULIFLOWER, SPINACH, AND CHEESE SOUP................. 128
235. CORNER-FILLING SOUP 128
236. LEMON GREEK SALAD 129
237. PEANUT SOUP... 129
238. ARTICHOKE SOUP 130
239. CURRIED PUMPKIN SOUP 130
240. CHEESY ONION SOUP 131

241. CREAM OF POTATO SOUP 131
242. SWISS CHEESE AND BROCCOLI SOUP 132
243. TAVERN SOUP 132
244. BROCCOLI BLUE CHEESE SOUP 133
245. CREAM OF MUSHROOM SOUP 133
246. HEALTHY BROCCOLI SALAD....................................134
247. OLIVE SOUP 134
248. SALMON SOUP..135
249. LOADED POTATO SOUP...135
250. BUTTERNUT SQUASH, APPLE, BACON AND ORZO SOUP ...136
251. CHICKEN ENCHILADA SOUP 136
252. TEX-MEX CHICKEN TORTILLA SOUP...........................137
253. WHITE BEAN AND CABBAGE SOUP.............................137

CHAPTER 14. DESSERT RECIPES 138

254. YOGURT MINT 138
255. RICE PUDDING 138
256. BRAISED APPLES..139
257. WINE FIGS 139
258. CINNAMON BITES 140
259. SWEET CHAI BITES 140
260. LEMON CURD 141
261. RHUBARB DESSERT 141
262. RASPBERRY COMPOTE 142
263. POACHED PEARS 142
264. APPLE CRISP 143
265. TASTY BANANA CAKE 143
266. MINI LAVA CAKES 144
267. APPLE BREAD 144
268. CHOCOLATE ORANGE BITES....................................145
269. CARAMEL CONES..145
270. CHOCOLATE FONDUE 146
271. BANANA BREAD 146
272. BREAD PUDDING 147
273. WRAPPED PEARS 147
274. COCOA CAKE 148
275. FLUFFY BITES 148
276. STRAWBERRY CHEESECAKE MINIS 149

CHAPTER 15. FUELING HACKS RECIPES 150

277. BERRY MOJITO 150
278. VANILLA FRAPPÉ 150
279. VANILLA SHAKE 151
280. MAPLE PANCAKES 151
281. BROWNIE PUDDING CUPS 152
282. TIRAMISU SHAKE 152
283. POTATO BAGELS 153
284. TROPICAL SMOOTHIE BOWL 153
285. MOCHA CAKE 154
286. LITTLE FUDGE BALLS 154
287. BROWNIE COOKIES 155
288. ZUCCHINI SPAGHETTI 155
289. CABBAGE AND RADISHES MIX 156
290. FLAVORSOME WAFFLES 156
291. RICHLY TASTY CREPE 157
292. CRUNCHY COOKIES 157
293. DELICIOUS FRENCH TOAST STICKS............................158

294. SHAMROCK SHAKE 158
295. PUMPKIN WAFFLES 159
296. CHOCOLATE DONUTS... 159
297. CHICKEN NUGGETS... 160
298. PEANUT BUTTER COOKIES.. 160
299. MINT COOKIES 161
300. PARMESAN ZUCCHINI ROUNDS 161
301. GREEN BEAN CASSEROLE 162

BONUS RECIPES...163

302. BANANA AND PUMPKIN WAFFLES 163
303. CHICKEN & ZUCCHINI PANCAKES............................. 163
304. DAMN BEST PORK CHOPS.. 164
305. MIXED VEGETABLE SOUP... 164
306. AIR-FRIED BANANAS... 165

307. GOLDEN TURMERIC FISH.. 165
308. SQUASH HASH 166
309. CHICKEN & VEGGIE QUICHE 166
310. CHIPOTLE PORK LOIN 167
311. CHICKEN WITH YELLOW SQUASH.............................. 167
312. JALAPENO GRILLED SALMON WITH TOMATO CONFIT 168
313. ZUCCHINI LEAN PORK BURGER 168
314. MINI ZUCCHINI BITES 169
315. BAKED CHICKEN & BELL PEPPERS 169

MEAL PLAN 5&1...170

MEAL PLAN 4&2&1 173

CONCLUSION 178

INTRODUCTION

This LEAN AND GREEN COOKBOOK provides you with delicious, healthy recipes easy to prepare using minimal or no oil. Leisure and physical activities were once considered necessary, but we hardly take time to exercise these days, and it isn't easy to find the time to organize fun activities. When we overeat, we often feel stressed and over-tired because we haven't rested in a while. This can also lead to serious health problems such as diabetes and high blood pressure.

So why would you need another cookbook that promotes healthy eating? The answer is simple: You never know when you might need it... when you feel like you are about to give in because of lack of willpower... when you just want to say 'Stop!' and give yourself a break... when you don't want to hit the ice cream and the cookies and the pizza again... when you feel like giving up.

This cookbook can be your secret weapon in making your life healthy, fun, and full of things that make you happy. It is not about eating an extremely low-fat diet (although it is possible to do so if you wish). Although some fantastic cookbooks provide meals that use virtually no oil or butter at all, this LEAN AND GREEN COOKBOOK takes a different approach: It provides recipes that use 1 to 3 tablespoons of fat per serving--not much at all (remember: 1 tbsp. = 15 ml). The recipes provide a delicious and decadent experience while still allowing you to feel great about what you're eating.

After so many years of eating whatever you wanted, eating healthy has become a chore. For some people, food is their best friend, and for others, it's one of their worst enemies. But after trying the recipes in this book, I guarantee you will be feeling happy and relaxed about your food... not defeated and stressed out!

And if nothing else, this cookbook can be used as a guide to inspire your own creations. It's meant to be an interactive guide that encourages you to try out different ingredients.

Once you have a collection of recipes at your disposal, it is simply a matter of combining them to create new meals. Remember, if you don't like something from one recipe, try another recipe from this book. If that doesn't work, try a different ingredient!

And if you find any of the recipes too intense for you, simply use less intense ingredients and/or lower your fat intake per serving. If you think it takes more than 1 tablespoon of oil or butter per serving to make it taste amazing, think again! You don't have to eat as much as you think you should because there are so many ways to add flavor without using so much fat. Remember: One tablespoon of oil is only 15 ml.

If this sounds like an easy diet, don't be fooled! I have been a vegetarian for over ten years, and I do not feel satisfied after eating very little. This is because everything has been processed, and our taste buds have been trained to want more. For me, eating a perfectly balanced meal is a challenge.

The recipes in this book are a joy to prepare and will help you feel more energized after eating! Once you get the hang of the various ingredients, I am sure you will find new techniques for preparing your favorite dishes!

CHAPTER 1.

WHAT IS A LEAN AND GREEN DIET?

In short, the Lean and Green diet basis is a reduced carb program that combine processed, packaged calorie-counted foods with homemade meals which encourage weight loss. You can choose from several options. All include products called "fuelings" as well as homemade meals, which follow the Lean and Green carb-fat ratio. The fuelings comprise over sixty items low in carbs, but high in protein and probiotic cultures. These friendly bacteria can boost your gut health and they include snack bars, cookies, shakes, puddings, cereals, soups, and pasta. All super-convenient and nutritious, while designed to help you feel satisfied.

What Do You Eat on a Lean and Green Diet?

It's the first question that people always ask about a new diet: "What will I be eating?" Because food is important to us all. It is not only essential to our life, but it is also pleasurable and sociable. Most of us are used to eating a range of foods from all the essential groups, but we all have to confess that we have our favorites, and our pet hates! So, firstly, let me reassure you, by telling you what you won't be eating: there is nothing in the Lean and Green diet that is "weird", unusual or just boring and unappetizing! You will be eating a huge selection of natural, nourishing foods; foods that you are already used to preparing and eating. The weight-loss secret lies in the planning, support, and execution of the program that you will be choosing to suit your needs and preferences. The Lean and Green diet plan includes two weight loss programs, in addition to a carefully balanced weight maintenance plan. To answer this question: what you eat, how frequently you eat it, and how much of it you will be eating, depends totally on the plans you choose, and at which stage of the plan you are on at any given time. A lot of diets on the market are successful only because they radically limit the types of food that you are allowed to eat, and how you are able to cook or combine them. Lean and Green doesn't do this, because we think that this way to eat can become rather boring eventually. Now you don't have to worry about that; there are no unpleasant surprises in store when you choose to eat Lean and Green! The wide variety and the numerous styles of food that you will be enjoying will keep you feeling nourished and happy to continue. This specialized cookbook will help you to prepare and include all of the readily available, low-cost, popular foods which should always appear in any healthy diet. What's more, using Lean and Green, you will be eating a lot of familiar, nourishing, scrummy foods at selected intervals throughout the day, which will help you to enrich your body while you are losing excess unhealthy weight. You will still be able to eat those lovely lean cuts of your favorite meats, like chicken, pork and beef. No limits on the amounts of greens and non-starchy vegetables that you consume either. You can tuck into the cabbage, kale, cauliflower, broccoli, asparagus, and zucchini. You are not limited to fat-free food either. On this diet, you will be eating tasty foods which contain healthy fats. Fats like olive and nut oil for cooking and salad dressing are good. If you are not vegan, you will be able to eat lots of low-fat dairy foods. Yummy yogurts and tasty cheeses are not off-limits! Fresh eggs, low-fat milk and frozen desserts are OK too. Lots of lovely fresh fruits are OK. Thumbs up to crisp apples, juicy oranges, sweet, grapes, zesty pineapples, and energizing bananas! Finally, to keep you feeling satisfied throughout the day, the Lean and Green diet naturally includes those comforting, life-giving, delicious essential whole grains and seeds. It's all well-balanced, convenient, and it tastes good!

What is Fueling?

Fueling is a measured, calorie-controlled way of snacking, and it helps you to maintain your energy levels, as well as feeling full throughout the day. More specifically, regular fuelings ensure that you are correctly nourished for your activity levels, whether you are working at your job, or working out. Correctly consumed fuelings provide you with the assurance that you won't be losing essential muscle mass while you are on the Lean and Green diet, because with carefully prepared fueling products, you'll be eating lots of protein, fiber and key nutrients, which are essential to sustaining muscle mass.

Foods to Avoid

When you eat more healthily, there are foods that you need to cut out. It's the usual suspects: fats should be the healthy kind; so, butter, vegetable shortening and coconut oil are not recommended. You should also limit the amounts of starchy vegetables you eat: corn, potatoes and peas, etc. Those with a sweet tooth: sugary drinks, desserts, cookies and chocolate are all out.

How Often Do You Eat on a Lean and Green Diet?

As you know, it's not what you eat or when you eat that's crucial to weight loss. How often you eat is also an important aspect. Lean and green is no exception to this rule. The eating habits and preferences that everyone has are as unique as their biology and personality. We are all creatures of habit. Some of our habits are good and some not so good! Some people enjoy eating at least one large meal every day, but they don't refuel in between times. They start their day with a hearty breakfast and eat frugally throughout the day. Some skip breakfast altogether, then have a quick snack for lunch, because they prefer to eat their main meal later. Some busy people are "grazers" who like to eat small, frequent meals. There is one group of people who snack all day long and never eat a balanced meal. Eating habits, and preferences for certain foods are totally personal. There are carb-loaders, there are sugar cravers, some are into fatty foods, and some are more health-conscious, following plant-based diets. Some people have to adjust their habits when they go Lean and Green. As I explained, the essence of the Lean and Green diet is to "fuel" your body regularly throughout the day, in order to supplement either one, two or three main meals. The simplicity and versatility of the Lean and Green diet is really helpful. You can try out all three plans, to see which one best meets your needs, and continues to work well for you over time. Once you reach your target weight, you can experiment. The cookbook will help you to do this, because it gives you recipes to prepare when you want to eat balanced, fresh food. The Lean and Green diet advises that you eat six or seven times per day depending on the plan.

Optimal Weight 5 & 1 Plan

This is the most popular plan, it includes five fuelings, and one balanced Lean and Green meal each day.

Optimal Weight 4 & 2 & 1 Plan

This is for people who need more calories and flexibility in food choices. This includes four fuelings, two Lean and Green meals, and one snack per day.

Optimal Health 3 & 3 Plan

This is specially designed for maintenance. It includes three fuelings and three balanced Lean and Green meals per day.

How Does Lean and Green Diet Work for Weight Loss?

The Lean and Green diet will work for you and support you if you want to lose excess weight and body fat and maintain the changes. One of the main reasons that the Lean and Green diet does work so efficiently is that the diet plan is so easy to implement and maintain, so you don't "fall off the wagon" and cheat yourself, by eating more than you should or foods that you shouldn't eat. The Lean and Green diet helps you to lose weight and cut your body fat because it is designed very precisely, to help you to get rid of those unwanted extra inches quickly. It helps you achieve this by reducing the calories and carbs you eat every day, through the use of the carefully portion-controlled meals and snacks included in the program. If you are using these meals and snacks and combine them with a regular exercise regime, (and you are not cheating and snacking on chocolate!) the end result will be a substantial overall weight loss and improved health that you can easily maintain.

Over the last twenty years, weight loss has become an influential industry, with many diets and products on the market. So, necessarily, there has been a lot of clinical research into the efficiency and safety of weight loss products and diets. Some studies have clearly shown that greater weight loss is ensured if those who wish to lose weight follow a regime that contains either full or partial meal replacement plans, compared with more traditional calorie-restricted diets which do not contain any meal replacement products.

The bottom line is that by reducing your overall calorie intake, the Lean and Green diet is going to be very effective for weight loss. If you follow the Lean and Green diet, as per the recommendations, it makes changing your eating habits very easy to do. A comprehensive sixteen-week study of 198 people confirmed that the people who were on the Lean and Green 5 & 1 Plan had significantly lower weight, and body fat, as well as smaller waist circumferences, compared with the people who were in the control group, who were not on the Lean and Green diet. Most people on the 5 & 1 Plan lost 5.7% of their body weight, though 28.1% lost 10%.

Give the Lean and Green diet a try. Using this supporting cookbook, the only thing that you have to lose is weight!

CHAPTER 2.

WHAT ARE THE BENEFITS OF THE LEAN AND GREEN DIET?

If you want a diet program simple and easy to execute, which can help you lose weight quickly, and provides built-in support networks, Lean and Green's plan may be a good match for you.

Easy to Follow

Since the diet depends primarily on pre-packaged foods, on the 5&1 plan, you are only accountable for preparing one meal a day. What is more, to make things easy to execute, each schedule arrives with food journals and sample food choices. Although you are expected to prepare 1-3 Lean and Green recipes every day, they are quick to create based on the plan since the package provides unique recipes and a selection of food choices. Besides, to supplement lean and green foods, many that are not interested in preparing can purchase prepared meals named "Flavors of Home."

The shakes, soups, and other such meal replacement items from Optavia are shipped straight to your house, a degree of comfort that is not offered by many other diets. While for "lean and green" dishes, you would need to look for your products, the home delivery alternative for the "Fuelings" of Lean and Green saves time and effort. They're quick to cook and make great grab-and-go dishes once the package arrives.

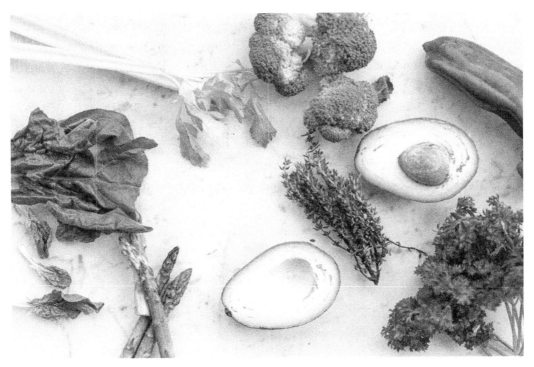

May Improve Blood Pressure

Via weight loss and decreased sodium intake, Lean and Green plans may help improve blood pressure. Although the Lean and Green diet has not been studied, a 40-week report on a related Medifast regimen in 90 individuals with extra weight or obesity showed a substantial decrease in blood pressure. Also, all Optavia meal plans are planned to have less than 2,300 milligrams of sodium a day, but it is up to you to use low sodium Lean and Green meal alternatives. Numerous health associations recommend drinking fewer than 2,300 mg of sodium a day, including the American Heart Association, College of Medicine, and the United States Department of Agriculture (USDA). That's because greater sodium consumption in sensitive populations is correlated with an elevated risk of hypertension and heart failure.

It Offers Continuous Support

For each weight-reduction plan, social support is a critical component of progress. The coaching service and community calls from Optavia include built-in motivation and customer assistance. Throughout weight reduction and maintenance plans, Lean and Green's fitness trainers are available. Specifically, one analysis identified a significant association between the amount of Lean and green 5&1 Strategy coaching sessions and enhanced weight loss. Also, evidence shows that long-term weight management is facilitated by obtaining a health coach or therapist. Coaching and community help is always excellent. Lean and Green provides coaching assistance and internet forums, video calls, and group meetings weekly. Training can be completely virtual, both digitally and by phone, but Lean and Green has a collection of coaches identified by area if you want to speak with a trainer in person.

Achieves Fast Weight Loss

To sustain their weight, most stable individuals consume about 1600 to 3000 calories a day. For specific individuals, reducing the amount to as little as 800 calories ensures weight reduction. The 5 & 1 strategy of Lean and Green is meant for accelerated weight loss, making it a healthy choice for those with a legitimate excuse to shed pounds quickly.

It Removes Guesswork

Some people learn that the most daunting aspect of healthy eating is the personal work needed to determine what to consume every day or even every dinner. Lean and Green alleviates the burden of meal preparation and "decision fatigue" by delivering "Fuelings" and "lean and green" menu suggestions to users for clear-cut accepted foods.

CHAPTER 3.

BREAKFAST RECIPES

1. Oatmeal Yogurt

Serving: 1
Difficulty: 1
Preparation Time: 5 minutes
Cooking Time: 5 minutes
Optavia Counts: 1 lean/ 0 green/ 0 healthy fats/ 0 condiments
Ingredients:

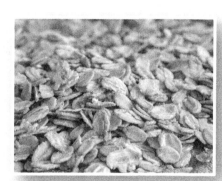

- ⅔ cup Greek-style yogurt
- 5 tsp. oatmeal
- ½ cup fresh persimmon
- 6 tsp. water

Directions:

1. Put the oatmeal in the pan.
2. Toast them, stirring constantly, until golden brown.
3. Then put them on a plate and let them cool down briefly.
4. Peel the persimmon and put it in a bowl with the water. Mix the whole thing into a fine puree.
5. Put the yogurt, the toasted oatmeal and then puree in layers in a glass and serve.

Nutrition: Calories: 286 kcal; Protein: 1 g; Fat: 11 g; Carbs: 29 g.

2. Muesli Smoothie Bowl

Serving: 1
Difficulty: 1
Preparation Time: 10 minutes
Cooking Time: 0 minutes
Optavia Counts: 0 lean/ 1 green/ 1 healthy fats/ 0 condiments
Ingredients:

- ⅔ cup yogurt
- 2 tbsp. apple
- 2 tbsp. mango
- 2 tbsp. low carb muesli
- 2 ½ tsp. spinach
- 2 ½ tsp. chia seeds

Directions:

1. Soak the spinach leaves and let them drain.
2. Peel the mango and cut it into strips.
3. Remove the apple core and cut it into pieces.
4. Put everything, except the mango, together with the yogurt in a blender and make a fine puree out of it.
5. Put the spinach smoothie in a bowl.
6. Add the muesli, chia seeds, and mango.
7. Serve the whole thing

Nutrition: Calories: 362 kcal; Protein: 12 g; Fat: 21 g; Carbs: 21 g.

3. Fried Egg with Bacon

Serving: 1
Difficulty: 1
Preparation Time: 5 minutes
Cooking Time: 10 minutes
Optavia Counts: 1 lean/ 0 green/ 1 healthy fats/ 2 condiments
Ingredients:

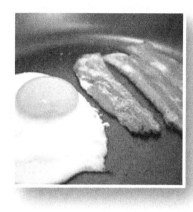

- 2 eggs
- 2 tbsp. of bacon
- 2 tbsp. olive oil
- Salt
- Pepper

Directions:

1. Heat oil in the pan and fry the bacon.
2. Reduce the heat and beat the eggs in the pan.
3. Cook the eggs and season with salt and pepper.
4. Serve the fried eggs hot with the bacon.

Nutrition: Calories: 405 kcal; Protein: 19 g; Fat: 38 g; Carbs: 1 g.

4. Grain Bread and Avocado

Serving: 1
Difficulty: 1
Preparation Time: 5 minutes
Cooking Time: 0 minutes
Optavia Counts: 1 lean/ 0 green/ 1 healthy fats/ 5 condiments
Ingredients:

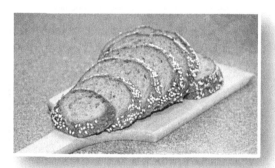

- 1 stick of thyme
- ½ lime
- ½ cup cottage cheese
- ½ avocado
- 2 slices whole meal bread
- Chili flakes
- Salt
- Black pepper

Directions:

1. Cut the avocado in half.
2. Remove the pulp and cut it into slices.
3. Pour the lime juice over it.
4. Wash the thyme and shake it dry.
5. Remove the leaves from the stem.
6. Brush the whole wheat bread with cottage cheese.
7. Place the avocado slices on top.
8. Top with chili flakes and thyme.
9. Add salt and pepper and serve.

Nutrition: Calories: 490 kcal; Protein: 19 g; Fat: 21 g; Carbs: 31 g.

5. Porridge with Walnuts

Serving: 1
Difficulty: 1
Preparation Time: 5 minutes
Cooking Time: 10 minutes
Optavia Counts: 0 lean/ 0 green/ 2 healthy fats/ 3 condiments
Ingredients:

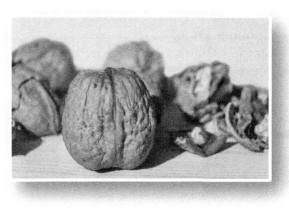

- 2 ½ tsp. of oatmeal
- ½ cup blueberries
- ½ tsp. cinnamon
- 5 tsp. crushed flaxseed
- ¼ cup ground walnuts
- 7 oz. nut drink
- ½ cup raspberries
- Agave syrup
- Salt

Directions:

1. Warm the nut drink in a small saucepan. Add the walnuts, flaxseed, and oatmeal, stirring constantly.
2. Stir in the cinnamon and salt.
3. Simmer for 8 minutes.
4. Keep stirring everything.
5. Sweet the whole thing.
6. Put the porridge in a bowl.
7. Wash the berries and let them drain.
8. Add them to the porridge and serve everything.

Nutrition: Calories: 378 kcal; Protein: 18 g; Fat: 27 g; Carbs: 11 g.

6. Mango Granola

Serving: 1
Difficulty: 1
Preparation Time: 10 minutes
Cooking Time: 30 minutes
Optavia Counts: 0 lean/ 0 green/ 5 healthy fats/ 3 condiments
Ingredients:

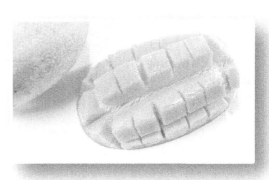

- 2 cups rolled oats
- 1 cup dried mango, chopped
- ½ cup almonds, roughly chopped
- ½ cup nuts
- ½ cup dates, roughly chopped
- 3 tbsp. sesame seeds
- 2 tsp. cinnamon
- 2 cups agave nectar
- 2 tbsp. coconut oil
- 2 tbsp. water

Directions:

1. Set the oven at 320°F.
2. In a large bowl, put the oats, almonds, nuts, sesame seeds, dates, and cinnamon, then mix well.
3. Meanwhile, heat a saucepan over medium fire, pour in the agave syrup, coconut oil, and water.
4. Stir and let it cook for at least 3 minutes or until the coconut oil has melted.
5. Gradually pour the syrup mixture into the bowl with the oats and nuts and stir well, ensure that all the ingredients are coated with the syrup. Transfer the granola to a baking sheet lined with parchment paper and place it in the oven to bake for 20 minutes.
6. After 20 minutes, take off the tray from the oven and lay the chopped dried mango on top. Put it back in the oven, then bake again for another 5 minutes.
7. Let the granola cool to room temperature before serving or placing it in an airtight container for storage. The shelf life of the granola will last up to 2 to 3 weeks.

Nutrition: Calories: 434; Protein: 13.16 g; Fat: 28.3 g; Carbs: 55.19 g.

7. Blueberry & Cashew Waffles

Serving: 2
Difficulty: 1
Preparation Time: 15 minutes
Cooking Time: 4 to 5 minutes
Optavia Counts: 1 lean/ 0 green/ 2 healthy fats/ 6 condiments
Ingredients:

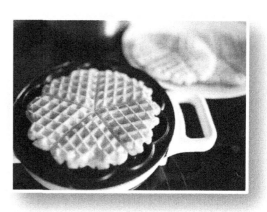

- 1 cup raw cashews
- 3 tbsp. coconut flour
- 1 tsp. baking soda
- Salt, to taste
- ½ cup unsweetened almond milk
- 3 organic eggs
- ¼ cup coconut oil, melted
- 3 tbsp. organic honey
- ½ tsp. organic vanilla flavor
- 1 cup fresh blueberries

Directions:

1. Preheat the waffle iron, and then grease it.
2. In a mixer, add cashews and pulse till flour-like consistency forms.
3. Transfer the cashew flour to a big bowl.
4. Add coconut flour, baking soda, and salt and mix well.
5. In another bowl, put the remaining ingredients and beat till well combined.
6. Put the egg mixture into the flour mixture, then mix till well combined.
7. Fold in blueberries.
8. In the preheated waffle iron, add the required amount of mixture.
9. Cook for around 4 to 5 minutes.
10. Repeat with the remaining mixture.

Nutrition: Calories: 432; Fat: 32 g; Carbs: 32 g; Protein: 13 g.

8. Eggless Scramble

Serving: 2
Difficulty: 1
Preparation Time: 10 minutes
Cooking Time: 8 minutes
Optavia Counts: 1 lean/ 3 green/ 1 healthy fats/ 3 condiments
Ingredients:

- 2 ¾ cup baby spinach
- ⅓ cup vegetable broth
- ¼ pound tofu
- 2 tsp. low-sodium soy sauce
- 1 garlic clove
- 1 tsp. turmeric
- 1 tbsp. olive oil
- 1 tsp. lemon juice

Directions:

1. Mince the garlic. Drain, press, and crumble the tofu.
2. In a frying pan, heat the olive oil over medium-high fire and sauté the garlic for about 1 minute.
3. Add the tofu and cook for about 2–3 minutes, slowly adding the broth.
4. Add the spinach, soy sauce, and turmeric, and stir fry for about 3–4 minutes or until all the liquid is absorbed.
5. Stir in the lemon juice and remove it from the heat.
6. Serve immediately.

Nutrition: Calories: 265 kcal; Protein: 14.89 g; Fat: 20.58 g; Carbs: 10.12 g.

9. Broccoli Waffles

Serving: 2
Difficulty: 1
Preparation Time: 10 minutes
Cooking Time: 8 minutes
Optavia Counts: 1 lean/ 1 green/ 1 healthy fat/ 4 condiments
Ingredients:

- ⅓ cup broccoli
- ½ tsp. dried onion
- 1 egg
- ¼ cup low-fat Cheddar cheese
- ½ tsp. garlic powder
- Salt
- Pepper

Directions:

1. Finely chop the broccoli.
2. Shred the cheddar and mince the onions.
3. Preheat a mini waffle iron and then grease it.
4. In a medium bowl, place all ingredients and mix until well combined.
5. Place ½ of the mixture into preheated waffle iron and cook for about 3-4 minutes or until golden brown. Repeat with the remaining mixture.
6. Serve warm.

Nutrition: Calories: 156 kcal; Protein: 10.59 g; Fat: 8.53 g; Carbs: 10.59 g.

10. Strawberry Yogurt Treats

Serving: 2
Difficulty: 1
Preparation Time: 10 minutes
Cooking Time: 0 minutes
Optavia Counts: 1 lean/ 0 green/ 2 healthy fat/ 1 condiments
Ingredients:

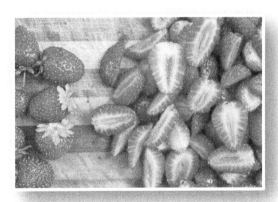

- 4 cups 0% fat plain Greek yogurt
- 1 cup strawberries
- 8 tbsp. of flax meal
- 4 tbsp. honey
- 8 tbsp. walnuts

Directions:

1. Chop the walnuts.
2. Wash and slice the strawberries.
3. Distribute 2 cups of the yogurt into your serving bowls.
4. Neatly layer the flax meal and the walnut in the middle.
5. Add a drizzle of half of the honey before covering it with the last layer of yogurt.
6. Add the honey on top of the yogurt to add color when you serve.

Nutrition: Calories: 733 kcal; Protein: 38.42 g; Fat: 30.57 g; Carbs: 83.44 g.

11. Apple Oatmeal

Serving: 2
Difficulty: 1
Preparation Time: 10 minutes
Cooking Time: 5 minutes
Optavia Counts: 0 lean/ 0 green/ 0 healthy fat/ 2 condiments
Ingredients:

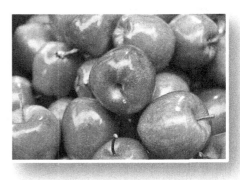

- 1 apple
- ⅔ cup rolled oats
- 1 cup water
- 1 cup any non-fat milk
- 1 tsp. ground cinnamon
- ¼ cup apple juice

Directions:

1. Peeled or unpeeled, chop the apple.
2. Place the water, juice, and apple in a deep pot. Bring to a boil over medium heat.
3. Add the oats and cinnamon. Bring to another boil. Lower the heat temperature and let it simmer for 3 minutes or until it is thick.
4. Divide the serving into two and serve with milk.

Nutrition: Calories: 277 kcal; Protein: 12.69 g; Fat: 7.69 g; Carbs: 52.71 g.

12. Kale Scramble

Serving: 2
Difficulty: 1
Preparation Time: 10 minutes
Cooking Time: 6 minutes
Optavia Counts: 1 lean/ 1 green/ 1 healthy fat/ 4 condiments
Ingredients:

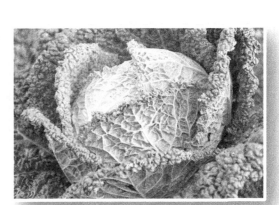

- 1 cup kale
- ⅛ tsp. ground turmeric
- ⅛ tsp. red pepper flakes
- 4 eggs
- 1 tbsp. water
- 2 tsp. olive oil
- Salt
- Black Pepper

Directions:

1. Crush the pepper flakes.
2. Remove the ribs and chop the kale.
3. In a bowl, add the eggs, turmeric, red pepper flakes, salt, pepper, and water and whisk until foamy.
4. In a skillet, heat the oil over medium fire.
5. Add the egg mixture and stir to combine.
6. Immediately reduce the heat to medium-low and cook for about 1-2 minutes, stirring frequently.
7. Stir in the kale and cook for about 3-4 minutes, stirring frequently.
8. Remove from the heat and serve immediately.

Nutrition: Calories: 314 kcal; Protein: 18.8 g; Fat: 23.91 g; Carbs: 5.27 g.

13. Cheesy Flax and Hemp Seeds Muffins

Serving: 2
Difficulty: 2
Preparation Time: 5 minutes
Cooking Time: 30 minutes
Optavia Counts: 1 lean/ 1 green/ 3 healthy fats/ 6 condiments
Ingredients:

- ¼ cup cottage cheese, low-fat
- ¼ cup raw hemp seeds
- ¼ cup almond meal
- ⅛ cup flax seeds meal
- ¼ tsp. baking powder
- 3 eggs
- ⅛ cup nutritional yeast flakes
- ¼ cup parmesan cheese
- ¼ cup scallion
- Salt
- 1 tbsp. olive oil

Directions:

1. Switch on the oven, then set it at 360°F and let it preheat. Meanwhile, take two ramekins, grease them with oil, and set them aside until required. Take a medium bowl, add flax seeds, hemp seeds, and almond meal. Then stir in salt and baking powder until mixed.
2. Crack eggs in another bowl. Add yeast, cottage cheese, and parmesan. Stir well until combined, and then stir this mixture into the almond meal mixture until incorporated.
3. Thinly slice the scallions. Fold them in, and then distribute the mixture between prepared ramekins and bake for 30 minutes until muffins are firm and the top is nicely golden brown.
4. When done, take out the muffins from the ramekins and let them cool completely on a wire rack.
5. For meal prepping, wrap each muffin with a paper towel and refrigerate for up to thirty-four days.
6. When ready to eat, reheat muffins in the microwave until hot and then serve.

Nutrition: Calories: 179 kcal; Protein: 15.4 g; Fat: 10.9 g; Carbs: 6.9 g.

14. Cheddar Broccoli Bread

Serving: 3
Difficulty: 3
Preparation Time: 15 minutes
Cooking Time: 45 minutes
Optavia Counts: 1 lean/ 1 green/ 2 healthy fats/ 3 condiments
Ingredients:

- ¼ cup shredded reduced-fat cheddar
- 3 cups small broccoli florets
- 1 tsp. cayenne pepper
- 4 eggs
- 1 tsp. black pepper
- ½ cup unsweetened almond milk
- Salt, to taste

Directions:

1. Preheat the oven to 375°F. Add 2 tablespoons of water and broccoli in a microwave-safe bowl and microwave it for about 4 minutes.
2. Take out and strain the broccoli. Meanwhile, add black pepper, cayenne pepper, salt, eggs, and almond milk in a large bowl. Beat well.
3. In a greased baking dish, arrange broccoli in the bottom and sprinkle cheese on it.
4. Pour the egg mixture on broccoli and cheese and bake for about 45 minutes.
5. Take out, slice, and serve.

Serving Suggestions: Serve with tea.
Variation Tip: You can also use mozzarella cheese for an even better taste.
Nutrition: Calories: 653; Fat: 36.9 g; Sat Fat: 2.2 g; Carbs: 24 g; Fiber: 9.2 g; Sugar: 0.5 g; Protein: 57.2 g.

15. Pomegranate, Nuts and Chia

Serving: 3
Difficulty: 1
Preparation Time: 5 minutes
Cooking Time: 10 minutes
Optavia Counts: 0 lean/ 0 green/ 5 healthy fats/ 2 condiments
Ingredients:

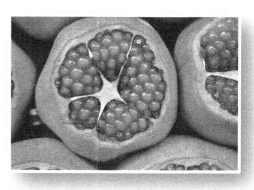

- ¼ cup hazelnuts
- ¼ cup walnuts
- ½ cup almond milk
- 4 tbsp. chia seeds
- 4 tbsp. pomegranate seeds
- 1 tsp. agave syrup
- Lime juice

Directions:

1. Finely chop the nuts.
2. Mix the almond milk with the chia seeds.
3. Let everything soak for 10 to 20 minutes.
4. Occasionally stir the mixture with the chia seeds.
5. Stir in the agave syrup.
6. Pour 2 tablespoons of each mixture into a dessert glass. Layer the chopped nuts on top.
7. Cover the nuts with 1 tablespoon each of the chia mass.
8. Sprinkle the pomegranate seeds on top and serve everything.

Nutrition: Calories: 248 kcal; Protein: 1 g; Fat: 19 g; Carbs: 7 g.

16. Bacon and Brussels Sprout Breakfast

Serving: 3
Difficulty: 1
Preparation Time: 10 minutes
Cooking Time: 15 minutes
Optavia Counts: 1 lean/ 1 green/ 2 healthy fats/ 5 condiments
Ingredients:

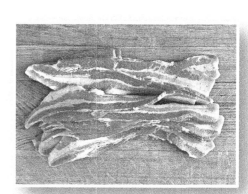

- 1 ½ tbsp. apple cider vinegar
- Salt
- 2 minced shallots
- 2 minced garlic cloves
- 3 medium eggs
- 12 oz. sliced Brussels sprouts
- Black pepper
- 2 oz. chopped bacon
- 1 tbsp. melted butter

Directions:

1. Over medium heat, quickly fry the bacon until crispy; then reserve on a plate.
2. Set the pan on fire again to fry garlic and shallots for 30 seconds.
3. Stir in apple cider vinegar, Brussels sprouts, and seasoning to cook for 5 minutes.
4. Add the bacon to cook for 5 minutes; then stir in the butter and set a hole at the center.
5. Crash the eggs to the pan and let cook fully. Enjoy!

Nutrition: Calories: 275 kcal; Protein: 17.4 g; Fat: 16.5 g; Carbs: 17. 2 g.

17. Blueberry Moss Pancakes

Serving: 3
Difficulty: 1
Preparation Time: 6 minutes
Cooking Time: 20 minutes
Optavia Counts: 1 lean/ 1 green/ 3 healthy fats/ 1 condiments
Ingredients:

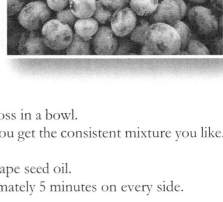

- 2 tbsps. grape seed oil
- 1 cup coconut milk
- ½ cup blueberries
- ½ cup alkaline water
- ½ cup agave
- 2 cups spelled flour
- ¼ tsp. sea moss

Directions:

1. Mix the spelled flour, agave, grape seed oil, hemp seeds, and sea moss in a bowl.
2. Add in 1 cup of hemp milk and alkaline water to the mixture until you get the consistent mixture you like.
3. Crimp the blueberries into the batter.
4. Heat the skillet to moderate fire, and then lightly coat it with the grape seed oil.
5. Pour the batter into the skillet, and then let them cook for approximately 5 minutes on every side.
6. Serve and enjoy.

Nutrition: Calories: 203 kcal; Protein: 4.8 g; Fat: 1.4 g; Carbs: 41.6 g.

18. Banana Cashew Toast

Serving: 3
Difficulty: 1
Preparation Time: 10 minutes
Cooking Time: 0 minutes
Optavia Counts: 0 lean/ 0 green/ 2 healthy fats/ 1 condiments
Ingredients:

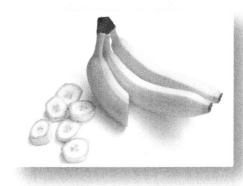

- 2 ripe medium-sized bananas
- 1 cup roasted cashews
- Cinnamon
- 2 tsp. flax meals
- 4 pieces oat bread
- 2 tsp. honey
- Salt

Directions:

1. Peel and slice the bananas.
2. Toast the bread.
3. In a food processor, puree the salt and cashews until they are smooth. Use the puree as a spread on the toasts.
4. On top of the spread, arrange a layer of bananas.
5. Add flax meals and a dash of cinnamon on top of the bananas.
6. Top the toast with honey.

Nutrition: Calories: 634 kcal; Protein: 13.42 g; Fat: 47.6 g; Carbs: 48.02 g.

19. Eggs and Avocado Toast

Serving: 4
Difficulty: 1
Preparation Time: 15 minutes
Cooking Time: 4 minutes
Optavia Counts: 1 lean/ 0 green/ 2 healthy fats/ 3 condiments
Ingredients:

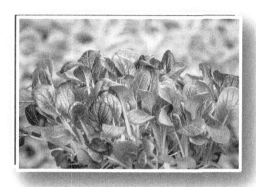

- 4 whole-wheat bread slices
- 4 hard-boiled eggs
- ¼ tsp. lemon juice
- 1 avocado
- Salt
- Ground black pepper

Directions:

1. Pit the avocado, then peel and chop it. Do the same with the eggs
2. In a bowl, add the avocado, and with a fork, mash it.
3. Combine lemon juice, pepper, and salt in a bowl and set aside.
4. Using a nonstick frying pan, on medium-high heat, toast the slices for about 2 minutes per side.
5. Spread the avocado mixture over each slice evenly. Top each with egg slices and serve immediately.

Nutrition: Calories: 162 kcal; Protein: 7.52 g; Fat: 12.69 g; Carbs: 5.93 g.

20. Cheesy Spinach Waffles

Serving: 4
Difficulty: 1
Preparation Time: 10 minutes
Cooking Time: 20 minutes
Optavia Counts: 1 lean/ 1 green/ 3 healthy fats/ 3 condiments
Ingredients:

- 4 oz. frozen spinach
- ½ cup part-skim Mozzarella cheese
- 1 large egg
- 1 cup ricotta cheese
- ¼ cup low-fat grated Parmesan cheese
- 1 garlic clove
- Salt
- Pepper

Directions: Crumble the ricotta cheese. Shred the mozzarella. Mince the garlic

1. Preheat a mini waffle iron and then grease it.
2. In a bowl, add all the ingredients and beat until well combined.
3. Place ¼ of the mixture into preheated waffle iron and cook for about 4-5 minutes or until golden brown. Repeat with the remaining mixture. Serve warm.

Nutrition: Calories: 178 kcal; Protein: 12.49 g; Fat: 11.82 g; Carbs: 6.14 g.

21. Swiss Chard and Spinach with Egg

Serving: 4
Difficulty: 1
Preparation Time: 5 minutes
Cooking Time: 10 minutes
Optavia Counts: 1 lean/ 3 green/ 1 healthy fat/ 3 condiments
Ingredients:

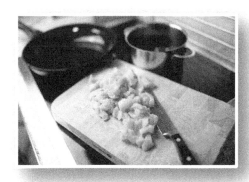

- 20 pieces Swiss chard leaves
- 4 pieces of rice bread
- 20 pieces spinach leaves
- 4 tbsp. parsley
- 4 egg whites
- 1 tsp. olive oil
- Salt
- Pepper
- Dried mint

Directions:

1. Bring to a boil 2 cups of water in a pan just below the boiling point. Open an egg; separate the whites from the yolks. Put the whites in a small bowl. Lower the bowl towards the heated water, and gently pour the egg into the pan. Do the same with the other eggs. Poach the eggs for 4 minutes.
2. After that, gently take the eggs one at a time and transfer them to a plate.
3. Do the same with the remaining 2 eggs. Chop the parsley and sauté the leaves in a pan for 6 minutes.
4. Toast the bread while doing this. When done, make a layer of the sautéed greens and chopped parsley on top of the toasted rice bread. Put the poached eggs above the bed of greens. Sprinkle each serving with ground pepper, sea salt, and dried mint.

Nutrition: Calories: 49 kcal; Protein: 5.31 g; Fat: 2.73 g; Carbs: 0.48 g.

22. Avocado Chicken Salad

Serving: 4
Difficulty: 1
Preparation Time: 5 minutes
Cooking Time: 10 minutes
Optavia Counts: 1 lean/ 0 green/ 2 healthy fat/ 5 condiments
Ingredients:

- 10 oz. diced cooked chicken
- ½ cup 2% plain Greek yogurt
- 3 oz. chopped avocado
- 12 tsp. garlic powder
- ¼ tsp. salt
- 1 tsp. pepper
- 1 tbsp. + 1 tsp. lime juice
- ¼ cup fresh cilantro, chopped

Directions:

1. Combine all ingredients in a medium-sized bowl. Refrigerate until ready to serve.
2. Cut the chicken salad in half and serve with your favorite greens.

Nutrition: Calories: 265; Protein: 35 g; Fat: 13 g; Carbs: 5 g.

23. Yogurt with Granola and Persimmon

Serving: 4
Difficulty: 1
Preparation Time: 5 minutes
Cooking Time: 5 minutes
Optavia Counts: 0 lean/ 1 green/ 1 healthy fat/ 0 condiments
Ingredients:

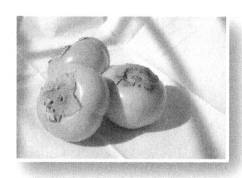

- 150 g. Greek-style yogurt
- 20 g. oatmeal
- 60 g. fresh persimmons
- 30 ml. of tap water

Directions:
1. Put the oatmeal in the pan without any fat.
2. Toast them, stirring constantly, until golden brown.
3. Then put them on a plate and let them cool down briefly.
4. Peel the persimmon and put it in a bowl with the water. Mix the whole thing into a fine puree.
5. Put the yogurt, the toasted oatmeal, and then puree in layers in a glass and serve.

Nutrition: Calories: 286; Carbs: 29 g; Protein: 1 g; Fat: 11 g.

24. Vegan-Friendly Banana Bread

Serving: 4
Difficulty: 3
Preparation Time: 15 minutes
Cooking Time: 40 minutes
Optavia Counts: 0 lean/ 0 green/ 1 healthy fat/ 7 condiments
Ingredients:

- 2 ripe bananas, mashed
- 1 cup brewed coffee
- 1 tbsp. chia seeds
- 6 tbsp. water
- ½ cup soft vegan butter
- ½ cup maple syrup
- 1 ¾ cups flour
- 2 tsp. baking powder
- 1 tsp. cinnamon powder
- 1 tsp. allspice
- ½ tsp. salt

Directions:
1. Set the oven at 350°F.
2. Bring the chia seeds in a small bowl, then soak them with 6 tablespoons of water. Stir well and set aside.
3. In a mixing bowl, mix the vegan butter and maple syrup using a hand mixer until it turns fluffy. Add the chia seeds along with the mashed bananas.
4. Mix well, and then add the coffee.
5. Meanwhile, sift all the dry ingredients (flour, baking powder, cinnamon powder, allspice, and salt) and then gradually add them into the bowl with the wet ingredients.
6. Combine the ingredients well, and then pour over a baking pan lined with parchment paper.
7. Place in the oven to bake for at least 30 to 40 minutes or until the toothpick comes out clean after inserting in the bread.
8. Allow the bread to cool before serving.

Nutrition: Calories: 371; Protein: 5.59 g; Fat: 16.81 g; Carbs: 49.98 g.

CHAPTER 4.

LUNCH RECIPES

25. Salmon Burgers

Serving: 1
Difficulty: 1
Preparation Time: 10 minutes
Cooking Time: 15 minutes
Optavia Counts: 1 lean/ 1 green/ 3 healthy fat/ 7 condiments
Ingredients:

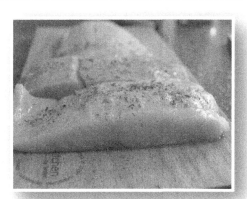

- pound salmon fillets
- 1 onion
- ¼ dill fronds
- 1 tbsp. honey
- 1 tbsp. horseradish
- 1 tbsp. mustard
- 1 tbsp. mayonnaise
- 1 tbsp. olive oil
- Toasted split rolls
- 1 avocado
- Salt and pepper, to taste
- Lettuce for serving

Directions:

1. Place salmon fillets in a blender and blend until smooth. Transfer to a bowl, add onion, dill, honey, horseradish and mix well. Add salt and pepper and form 4 patties.
2. In a bowl combine mustard, honey, mayonnaise, and dill in a skillet heat oil add salmon patties and cook for 2 to 3 minutes per side. When ready, remove from heat.
3. Divide lettuce and onion between the buns. Place salmon patty on top and spoon mustard mixture and avocado slices.
4. Serve when ready.

Nutrition: Calories: 180; Fat: 7 g; Carbs: 6 g; Protein: 12.8 g.

26. Stuffed Mushrooms

Serving: 1
Difficulty: 1
Preparation Time: 6 minutes
Cooking Time: 12 minutes
Optavia Counts: 0 lean/ 0 green/ 0 healthy fat/ 6 condiments
Ingredients:

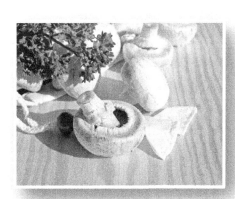

- 2 tsp. cumin powder
- 4 garlic cloves, peeled and minced
- 1 small onion, peeled and chopped
- 18 medium-sized white mushrooms
- Fine sea salt and freshly ground black pepper, to your liking
- A pinch ground allspice
- 1 tbsp. olive oil

Directions:

1. First, clean the mushrooms; remove the middle stalks from the mushrooms to prepare the "shells."
2. Grab a mixing dish and thoroughly combine the remaining items.
3. Fill the mushrooms with the prepared mixture.
4. Cook the mushrooms at 345°F and heat for 12 minutes. Enjoy!

Nutrition: Calories: 179; Fat: 14 g; Carbs: 8.8 g; Protein: 4.8 g.

27. Mini Mac in a Bowl

Serving: 1
Difficulty: 1
Preparation Time: 5 minutes
Cooking Time: 15 minutes
Optavia Counts: 1 lean/ 2 green/ 1 healthy fat/ 5 condiments
Ingredients:

- 5 oz. lean ground beef
- 2 tbsp. onion
- ⅛ tsp. onion powder
- ⅛ tsp. white vinegar
- 1 oz. dill pickle slices
- 1 tsp. sesame seed
- 1 cup romaine lettuce
- 1 tbsp. reduced-fat cheddar cheese
- 2 tbsp. thousand islands

Directions:

1. Place a lightly greased small pan on the fire and heat. Sautee the diced onion for about 2–3 minutes.
2. Then, add the beef and let it fry until brown. Next, mix the vinegar and onion powder with the dressing.
3. Finally, add the cooked meat on top of the shredded lettuce and sprinkle with cheese. Add the cucumber slices.
4. Drizzle with sauce and sprinkle the sesame seeds on top.

Nutrition: Calories: 646 kcal; Protein: 23.3 g; Fat: 55.9 g; Carbs: 12.4 g.

28. Zucchini Frittata

Serving: 1
Difficulty: 2
Preparation Time: 20 minutes
Cooking Time: 20 minutes
Optavia Counts: 0 lean/ 2 green/ 3 healthy fat/ 2 condiments
Ingredients:

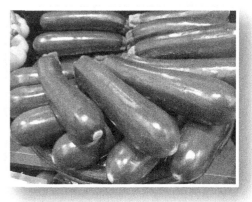

- 2 tbsp. oil
- 2 zucchinis
- 2 eggs
- 1 cup flour
- 1 tsp. baking powder
- ½ cup scallions
- Salt
- Black pepper

Directions:

1. Wash the zucchinis. Cut the ends off the zucchinis and grate them into a mixing bowl.
2. Stir in 1 teaspoon of salt and set aside for about 10 minutes.
3. Squeeze the grated zucchini dry to remove as much water as possible.
4. Add the two whole eggs and the chopped green onions.
5. In a bowl, combine 1 cup of flour, ½ teaspoon of salt, ½ teaspoon of black pepper, and 1 teaspoon of baking powder.
6. Then add the contents of the smaller bowl to the larger bowl with the grated zucchini.
7. Stir everything together; until it's well mixed.
8. Preheat a saucepan to medium heat and add two tablespoons of oil.
9. Add the zucchini mixture, a heaping tablespoon at a time.
10. Fry the mixture for about 4 minutes on each side until the mixture turns a golden-brown color.
11. Add more oil to the pan if needed.

Nutrition: Calories: 1082 kcal; Protein: 39.17 g; Fat: 50.01 g; Carbs: 122.85 g.

29. Chicken Omelet

Serving: 1
Difficulty: 1
Preparation Time: 5 minutes
Cooking Time: 15 minutes
Optavia Counts: 3 lean/ 1 green/ 2 healthy fat/ 3 condiments
Ingredients:

- 1 oz. rotisserie chicken; shredded
- 1 tsp. mustard
- 4 eggs
- 1 tbsp. mayonnaise
- 1 tomato
- 6 bacon slices
- 1 small avocado
- Sea salt
- Black pepper

Directions:

1. In a bowl, mix the eggs with a little salt and pepper and whisk.
2. Heat a skillet over medium fire; spray it with a little cooking oil, add the eggs, and fry your omelet for 5 minutes.
3. Add chicken, avocado, chopped tomato, cooked and crumbled bacon, mayo, and mustard to one-half of the omelet.
4. Fold the omelet, cover the pan and cook for another 5 minutes.
5. Transfer to a plate and serve.

Nutrition: Calories: 400 kcal; Protein: 25.6 g; Fat: 32.4 g; Carbs: 4.4 g.

30. Chicken Pesto Pasta

Serving: 1
Difficulty: 2
Preparation Time: 5 minutes
Cooking Time: 15 minutes
Optavia Counts: 2 lean/ 3 green/ 2 healthy fat/ 4 condiments
Ingredients:

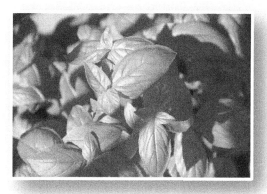

- 3 cups raw kale leaves
- 2 tbsp. olive oil
- 2 cups basil
- Salt
- 3 tbsp. lemon juice
- 3 garlic cloves
- 2 cups cooked chicken breast
- 1 cup baby spinach
- 6 oz. uncooked chicken pasta
- 1/8 oz. ball of fresh mozzarella
- Basil leaves
- Red pepper flakes

Directions:

1. Pesto: Put the kale, lemon juice, basil, garlic cloves, olive oil, and salt in a blender and puree until smooth. Season to taste with pepper.
2. Pasta: Boil the pasta and drain the water. Reserve ¼ cup of the liquid.
3. Take a bowl and mix everything, the cooked pasta, the pesto, the chicken cubes, the spinach, the mozzarella, and the reserved pasta liquid.
4. Sprinkle with chopped basil or red paper flakes. Serve warm or chilled.

Nutrition: Calories: 1206 kcal; Protein: 128.22 g; Fat: 50.2 g; Carbs: 61.8 g.

31. Crab Cakes

Serving: 2
Difficulty: 1
Preparation Time: 20 minutes
Cooking Time: 10 minutes
Optavia Counts: 2 lean/ 1 green/ 2 healthy fat/ 4 condiments
Ingredients:

- ½ pound lump crabmeat, drained
- 2 tbsp. coconut flour
- 1 tbsp. mayonnaise
- ¼ tsp. green Tabasco sauce
- 1 tbsp. butter
- 1 small egg, beaten
- ¾ tbsp. fresh parsley, chopped
- ½ tsp. yellow mustard
- Salt and black pepper, to taste

Directions:

1. Mix together all the ingredients in a bowl except butter.
2. Make patties from this mixture and set them aside.
3. Heat butter in a skillet over medium fire and add patties. Cook for about 10 minutes on each side and dish out to serve hot.
4. You can store the raw patties in the freezer for about 3 weeks for meal prepping.
5. Place patties in a container and place parchment paper in between the patties to avoid stickiness.

Nutrition: Calories: 153; Fat: 10 g; Carbs: 6.8 g.

32. Cayenne Rib Eye Steak

Serving: 2
Difficulty: 1
Preparation Time: 10 minutes
Cooking Time: 13 minutes
Optavia Counts: 1 lean/ 0 green/ 3 healthy fat/ 5 condiments
Ingredients:

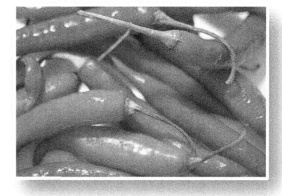

- 1-pound rib eye steak.
- 1 tsp. salt.
- 1 tsp. cayenne pepper.
- ½ tsp. chili flakes.
- 1 tbsp. cream.
- 1 tsp. olive oil.
- 1 tsp. lemongrass.
- 1 tbsp. butter.
- 1 tsp. garlic powder.

Directions:

1. Preheat the Air Fryer to 360°F. Take a shallow bowl and combine the cayenne pepper, salt, chili flakes, lemongrass, and garlic powder. Mix the spices gently. Sprinkle the rib eye steak with the spice mixture.
2. Melt the butter and combine it with cream and olive oil. Churn the mixture.
3. Pour the churned mixture into the Air Fryer basket tray. Add the rib eye steak.
4. Cook the steak for 13 minutes. Do not stir the steak during the cooking.
5. When the steak is cooked, transfer it to a paper towel to soak all the excess fat.
6. Serve the steak. You can slice the steak if desired.

Nutrition: Calories: 708; Fat: 59 g; Carbs: 2.3 g; Protein: 40.4 g.

33. Pasta with Avocado and Cream

Serving: 2
Difficulty: 1
Preparation Time: 10 minutes
Cooking Time: 6 minutes
Optavia Counts: 0 lean/ 0 green/ 2 healthy fat/ 3 condiments
Ingredients:
- ½ tsp. dried basil
- ⅛ cup heavy cream
- ½ avocado
- ½ pack of shirataki noodles, cooked
- Salt
- Black pepper

Directions:
1. Fill a medium saucepan halfway with water and bring to a boil over medium heat; then add pasta and cook for 2 minutes. Then drain the pasta and set aside until ready to use.
2. Put the avocado in a bowl and mash it with a fork. Transfer to a blender, add remaining ingredients and blend until smooth.
3. Take a pan, put it on medium heat and when it is hot, add the noodles. Pour in the avocado mixture, stir well and cook for 2 minutes until hot.
4. Serve immediately.

Nutrition: Calories: 131 kcal; Protein: 1.2 g; Fat: 12.6 g; Carbs: 4.9 g.

34. Spaghetti Squash with Cheese and Pesto

Serving: 2
Difficulty: 2
Preparation Time: 10 minutes
Cooking Time: 35 minutes
Optavia Counts: 1 lean/ 0 green/ 3 healthy fat/ 3 condiments
Ingredients:

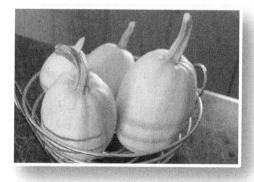

- 1 Cup cooked spaghetti squash
- Salt to taste
- Black pepper
- ½ tbsp. olive oil
- ¼ cup ricotta cheese
- 4 oz. fresh mozzarella cheese
- ⅛ cup basil pesto

Directions:
1. Preheat oven to 375°F.
2. Take a bowl, put the drained spaghetti squash in it and season it with salt and black pepper.
3. Using a baking dish, grease it with oil, put the squash mixture in it, cover it with ricotta cheese and cubed mozzarella and bake it for 10 minutes until cooked.
4. Drizzle pesto over and serve.

Nutrition: Calories: 169 kcal; Protein: 11.9 g; Fat: 11.3 g; Carbs: 6.2 g.

35. Eggs in Pepper Rings

Serving: 2
Difficulty: 1
Preparation Time: 10 minutes
Cooking Time: 6 minutes
Optavia Counts: 1 lean/ 1 green/ 0 healthy fat/ 4 condiments
Ingredients:

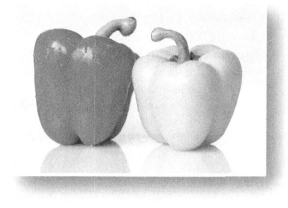

- 1 bell pepper
- 4 eggs
- 1 tbsp. parsley
- 1 tbsp. chives
- Salt
- Pepper

Directions:

1. Heat a lightly greased nonstick skillet over medium fire.
2. Cut the bell pepper into 4 rings.
3. Place 4 bell pepper rings in the skillet and cook for about 2 minutes.
4. Carefully flip the rings.
5. Crack an egg into the center of each pepper ring and sprinkle with salt and black pepper.
6. Fry for about 2-4 minutes or until the eggs have reached the desired doneness.
7. Carefully transfer the pepper rings to serving plates and serve garnished with chopped parsley and chopped chives.

Nutrition: Calories: 278 kcal; Protein: 18.94 g; Fat: 19.39 g; Carbs: 6.47 g.

36. Fish Lettuce Tacos

Serving: 2
Difficulty: 2
Preparation Time: 10-15 minutes
Cooking Time: 25-30 minutes
Optavia Counts: 1 lean/ 0 green/ 1 healthy fat/ 6 condiments
Ingredients:

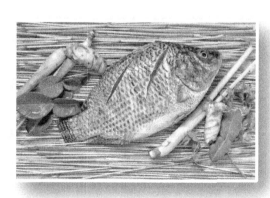

- ½ tsp. chili powder
- 20 oz. raw tilapia
- ½ tsp. ground cumin

Toppings:

- 2 tsp. lime juice
- 4 tbsp. dressing of choice
- 3 oz. avocado
- Salt
- Black pepper

Directions:

1. Preheat the oven to 375°F.
2. Line a baking sheet with parchment paper. Sprinkle both sides of the tilapia with salt, pepper, cumin and chili powder.
3. Bake for 20 to 25 minutes, or until cooked through.
4. Spoon some fish in a lettuce boat to hold it. Drizzle each serving with 1 teaspoon of lime juice and 2 tablespoons of dressing. Serve with avocado.

Nutrition: Calories: 68 kcal; Protein: 1 g; Fat: 6 g; Carbs: 3 g.

37. Meatball Lasagna

Serving: 2
Difficulty: 1
Preparation Time: 15 - 10 minutes
Cooking Time: 15-20 minutes
Optavia Counts: 1 lean/ 2 green/ 3 healthy fat/ 2 condiments
Ingredients:

- 4 tsp. grated parmesan cheese
- 2 cups zucchini
- ½ cup skim ricotta cheese
- ½ cup 2% mozzarella cheese
- 12 turkey meatballs
- ½ tsp. basil
- 1 cup tomatoes
- Garlic salt

Directions:

1. Preheat the oven to 350°F.
2. Layer zucchini slices in a medium-sized casserole dish. Spread ricotta cheese over the squash. Sprinkle garlic salt and basil over.
3. Mix diced tomatoes with meatballs in a bowl. Pour over ricotta cheese. Sprinkle mozzarella over meatballs and then top with grated parmesan cheese. Bake for 25 minutes or until cheese is melted.
4. Drain the water from the dish by tilting carefully. Serve.

Nutrition: Calories: 584 kcal; Protein: 46 g; Fat: 41 g; Carbs: 4 g.

38. Lettuce Salad with Beef Strips

Serving: 3
Difficulty: 1
Preparation Time: 10 minutes.
Cooking Time: 12 minutes.
Optavia Counts: 1 lean/ 2 green/ 3 healthy fat/ 5 condiments
Ingredients:

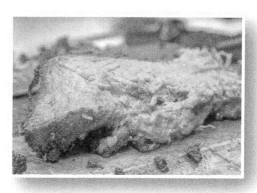

- 2 cups lettuce
- 10 oz. beef brisket
- 2 tbsp. sesame oil
- 1 tbsp. sunflower seeds
- 1 cucumber
- 1 tsp. ground black pepper
- 1 tsp. paprika
- 1 tsp. Italian spices
- 1 tsp. butter
- 1 tsp. dried dill
- 1 tbsp. coconut milk

Directions:

1. Cut the beef brisket into strips.
2. Sprinkle the beef strips with the ground black pepper, paprika, and dried dill.
3. Preheat the Air Fryer to 365°F.
4. Put the butter in the Air Fryer basket tray and melt it.
5. Then add the beef strips and cook them for 6 minutes on each side.
6. Meanwhile, tear the lettuce and toss it in a big salad bowl.
7. Crush the sunflower seeds and sprinkle them over the lettuce.
8. Chop the cucumber into the small cubes and add to the salad bowl.
9. Then combine the sesame oil and Italian spices together. Stir the oil.
10. Combine the lettuce mixture with the coconut milk and stir it using 2 wooden spatulas.
11. When the meat is cooked, let it chill to room temperature.
12. Add the beef strips to the salad bowl.
13. Stir it gently and sprinkle the salad with the sesame oil dressing.
14. Serve the dish immediately. **Nutrition: Calories:** 199 kcal; Fat: 12.4 g; Carbs: 3.9 g; Protein: 18.1 g.

39. Mozzarella, Tomatoes and Pesto Chicken

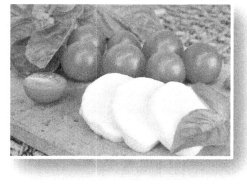

Serving: 3
Difficulty: 2
Preparation Time: 5-15 minutes
Cooking Time: 20-25 minutes
Optavia Counts: 1 lean/ 1 green/ 1 healthy fat/ 3 condiments
Ingredients:

- ½ cup part-skim mozzarella
- 1 cup tomato
- 4 tsp. pesto
- 16 oz. chicken breast
- Salt
- Pepper

Directions:

1. Cut chicken breast horizontally into 4 thinner cutlets. Season with salt and pepper.
2. Preheat the oven to 400°F. Line a baking sheet with parchment paper. Place the chicken and spread 1 teaspoon of pesto over. Bake 15 minutes or until chicken is no longer pink in the center.
3. Remove from oven, top with diced tomatoes, shredded mozzarella and parmesan cheese.
4. Bake for an extra 3 to 5 minutes or until cheese is melted.
5. Serve

Nutrition: Calories: 601 kcal; Protein: 59 g; Fat: 38 g; Carbs: 2 g.

40. Cheesy Jalapeños

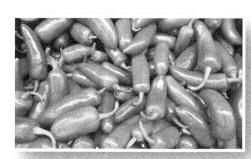

Serving: 3
Difficulty: 2
Preparation Time: 10-15 minutes
Cooking Time: 20-25 minutes
Optavia Counts: 0 lean/ 1 green/ 3 healthy fat/ 1 condiments
Ingredients:

- 2 light cream cheese triangles
- ¼ cup 2% reduced-fat Cheese Blend
- ⅛ tsp. Worcestershire sauce
- 3 to 4 jalapeños
- 1 tbsp. parmesan cheese

Directions:

1. Cut jalapenos in half lengthwise; remove seeds and membranes.
2. In a large saucepan, boil peppers in water for 5-10 minutes (the longer you boil the peppers, the milder they become). Drain and rinse in cold water; set aside. Preheat oven to 400°F.
3. In a small mixing bowl, beat the light cream cheese, cheddar cheese and Worcestershire sauce (optional).
4. Scoop 2 teaspoons into each jalapeño half; sprinkle with grated Parmesan cheese.
5. Place on a greased baking sheet. Bake at 400°F for 5-10 minutes or until the cheese is melted.
6. Serve warm.

Nutrition: Calories: 158 kcal; Protein: 10.3 g; Fat: 10.8 g; Carbs: 4.5 g.

41. Avocados Stuffed with Salmon

Serving: 3
Difficulty: 1
Preparation Time: 5 minutes
Cooking Time: 5 minutes
Optavia Counts: 1 lean/ 1 green/ 3 healthy fat/ 2 condiments
Ingredients:

- 2 oz. smoked salmon
- 2 tbsp. olive oil
- Lemon juice
- 1 avocado
- 1 oz. goat cheese
- Sea salt
- Pepper

Directions:

1. Combine the salmon, lemon juice, oil, cheese, salt and pepper in your food processor and pulse well.
2. Spread this mixture over the avocado halves and serve.

Nutrition: Calories: 300 kcal; Protein: 16.7 g; Fat: 15.1 g; Carbs: 8.8 g.

42. Chicken Gordon Bleu

Serving: 3
Difficulty: 3
Preparation Time: 5-10 minutes
Cooking Time: 25-30 minutes
Optavia Counts: 1 lean/ 1 green/ 3 healthy fat/ 2 condiments
Ingredients:

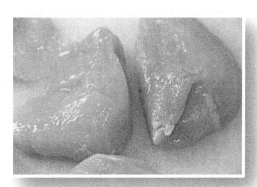

- ½ cup tomato
- 18 oz. boneless, skinless chicken breasts
- 4 oz. part-skim mozzarella cheese
- 2 cups spinach

Italian Dressing:

- 1 tbsp. Dijon Mustard
- 1 tbsp. white wine vinegar
- 1 packet Splenda
- 1 tsp. olive oil
- ½ tsp. Italian mixed herbs
- 3 cups red pepper flakes
- Sea salt
- Black pepper

Directions:

1. Preheat the oven to 350°F.
2. Whisk Italian dressing ingredients together in a bowl.
3. Cut a pocket in each chicken breast, being careful not to cut all the way through. Coat the chicken with the Italian Dressing, inside and outside.
4. Fill the chicken as much as you can with sun-dried tomato, top with cheese then finish with spinach leaves.
5. Seal using toothpicks.
6. Heat oil in a skillet over high fire. Add chicken and fry for 1 ½ minutes on each side, until golden brown.
7. Transfer to oven and cook for 15 minutes, until the cheese is melted and bubbly and chicken is cooked through.
8. Let rest for 3 minutes before serving, and drizzle with the juices from the pan.

Nutrition: Calories: 684 kcal; Protein: 135 g; Fat: 65 g; Carbs: 5 g.

43. Smoked Salmon with Avocado Oil

Serving: 3
Difficulty: 1
Preparation Time: 10 minutes
Cooking Time: 10 minutes
Optavia Counts: 2 lean/ 2 green/ 2 healthy fat/ 5 condiments
Ingredients:

- 4 eggs
- ½ tsp. avocado oil
- 4 oz. smoked salmon

For the Sauce:

- ½ cup cashews
- ¼ cup scallions
- 1 tsp. garlic powder
- 1 cup coconut milk
- 1 tbsp. lemon juice
- Sea salt
- Black pepper

Directions:

1. Place cashews in a blender with coconut milk, garlic powder, lemon juice and blend well.
2. Add salt, pepper, and chopped scallions. Blend well again, transfer to a bowl and store in the fridge.
3. Heat a frying pan with the oil over medium fire; add the eggs, whisk a little and fry until almost cooked.
4. Transfer to the preheated broiler and fry until the eggs are set.
5. Divide eggs among plates, top with smoked salmon and serve with scallion sauce on top.

Nutrition: Calories: 200 kcal; Protein: 15.1 g; Fat: 10.6 g; Carbs: 11.9 g.

44. Lemon Parmesan Salmon

Serving: 4
Difficulty: 2
Preparation Time: 10 minutes
Cooking Time: 25 minutes
Optavia Counts: 1 lean/ 2 green/ 2 healthy fat/ 2 condiments
Ingredients:

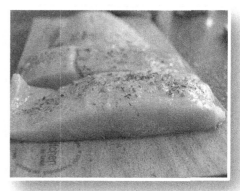

- ¼ pound salmon fillet
- ¼ tsp. thyme leaves dried
- 1 tbsp. scallions
- 1 tsp. grated lemon peel
- ¾ cup white breadcrumbs
- 2 tbsp. butter,
- ¼ tsp. salt
- ¼ cup grated parmesan cheese

Directions:

1. Preheat the oven to 350°F.
2. Mist cooking spray onto a baking pan. Fill with pat-dried salmon. Brush salmon with melted butter before sprinkling with salt.
3. Combine the breadcrumbs with chopped scallions, thyme, lemon peel, cheese, and remaining butter.
4. Cover salmon with the breadcrumb mixture. Air-fry for 15 to 25 minutes.

Nutrition: Calories: 290 kcal; Protein: 30 g; Fat: 10 g; Carbs: 0 g.

45. Tasty Pancakes

Serving: 4
Difficulty: 1
Preparation Time: 12 minutes
Cooking Time: 3 minutes
Optavia Counts: 1 lean/ 1 green/ 1 healthy fat/ 2 condiments
Ingredients:

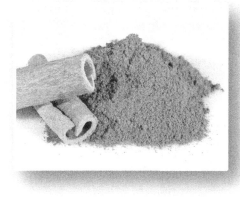

- 2 eggs
- 1 tsp. stevia
- 4 oz. cream cheese
- ½ tsp. cinnamon powder
- Cooking spray

Directions:

1. Place eggs in a blender with the cream cheese, stevia, cinnamon and blend well.
2. Heat skillet with spray over medium-high fire. Pour in ¼ of the batter, spread well, bake for 2 minutes, flip and bake for 1 minute more.
3. Transfer to a plate and repeat with the rest of the batter.
4. Serve immediately.

Nutrition: Calories: 344 kcal; Protein: 16.7 g; Fat: 23 g; Carbs: 3.7 g.

46. Tuna Cobbler

Serving: 4
Difficulty: 2
Preparation Time: 15 minutes
Cooking Time: 25 minutes
Optavia Counts: 1 lean/ 2 green/ 1 healthy fat/ 3 condiments
Ingredients:

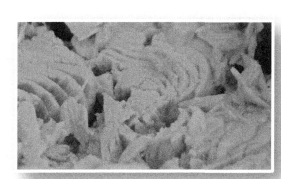

- 2 oz. hot peppers
- 10 oz. canned tuna
- 1 tsp. lemon juice
- ⅓ cup cold water
- 1 ½ cups mixed vegetables, frozen
- 10 ¾ oz. cream of chicken
- 1 tbsp. sweet pickle relish
- Paprika

Directions:

1. Preheat the Air Fryer at 375°F.
2. Mist cooking spray into a round casserole.
3. Mix the frozen vegetables with milk, cream, lemon juice, relish, sliced hot peppers, and tuna in a saucepan. Cook for 8 minutes over medium heat.
4. Fill the casserole with the mixture.
5. Mix the biscuit mixture with cold water to make a soft dough. Beat for half a minute and then pour by spoonsful into the casserole.
6. Season with paprika.
7. Fry in the Air Fryer for 25 minutes.

Nutrition: Calories: 320 kcal; Protein: 20 g; Fat: 10 g; Carbs: 30 g.

47. Bacon Frittatawith Asparagus

Serving: 4
Difficulty: 2
Preparation Time: 20 minutes
Cooking Time: 20 minutes
Optavia Counts: 2 lean/ 1 green/ 0 healthy fat/ 2 condiments
Ingredients:

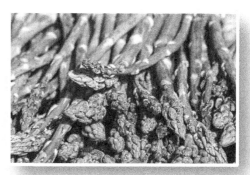

- 4 bacon slices
- Sea salt
- Black pepper
- 8 eggs
- Bunch asparagus

Directions:

1. Heat a frying pan, add crumbled bacon, stir and fry for 5 minutes.
2. Add cleaned and cut asparagus, salt and pepper, stir and cook for another 5 minutes.
3. Add the eggs, spread in the pan, place in oven and bake at 350°F for 20 minutes.
4. Divide and serve on plates.

Nutrition: Calories: 251 kcal; Protein: 7 g; Fat: 6 g; Carbs: 16 g.

48. Spaghetti Squash Casserole

Serving: 4
Difficulty: 4
Preparation Time: 20-25 minutes
Cooking Time: 100-120 minutes
Optavia Counts: 2 lean/ 1 green/ 4 healthy fat/ 3 condiments
Ingredients:

- 4 pounds spaghetti squash
- 8 oz. part-skim ricotta
- 8 oz. reduced-fat mozzarella cheese
- 2 tbsp. eggbeaters
- 2 tbsp. parmesan cheese
- 2 cups tomatoes
- ¼ tsp. garlic powder
- ⅛ tsp. salt
- ⅛ tsp. pepper
- 2 tsp. olive oil
- 6 oz. seasoned ground turkey

Directions:

1. Preheat oven to 400°F.
2. Prick squash with fork or metal skewer and roast in the oven for an hour or until it seems soft when you press on it. Then take it out and leave on the counter until cool.
3. When squash is cool, cut in half and scoop out the seeds and discard.
4. Use a fork or spoon to scoop out the rest of the squash and set it aside in a bowl.
5. Measure out 4 cups of spaghetti squash and store the rest in the fridge.
6. Add oil to a skillet over medium heat. Sauté the 4 cups of squash for a few minutes until it begins to brown. Then add garlic powder, salt and pepper if desired. Mix ricotta cheese, grated parmesan, eggbeaters and 4 oz. or 1 cup of mozzarella cheese together. Preheat oven to 375°F.
7. Pour 1 cup of the diced tomatoes on the bottom of a casserole dish and spread evenly.
8. Add squash. Top the squash with the ricotta cheese mixture. Then top the ricotta cheese mixture with the cooked ground turkey. Spread 1 cup of diced tomatoes over the meat. Bake for 35 minutes.
9. Spread the rest of the mozzarella cheese over the top and bake an additional 25 minutes until cheese is melted and lightly brown. Let rest for 10 minutes or so to serve.

Nutrition: Calories: 593 kcal; Protein: 39.6 g; Fat: 25.7 g; Carbs: 54.6 g.

CHAPTER 5.

SNACK RECIPES

49. Cauliflower Pizza with Chicken & Tzatziki

Servings: 1
Difficulty: 3
Preparation Time: 10 minutes
Cooking Time: 50 minutes
Optavia Counts: 2 lean/ 3 green/ 3 healthy fat/ 4 condiments
Ingredients:

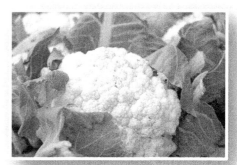

- 5 ½ cups Frozen Riced Cauliflower
- 2 large eggs
- 1 tbsp. low-fat parmesan cheese
- ¼ tbsp. salt divided (optional)
- 1 pound boneless skinless chicken breast sliced
- 10 large kalamata olives
- ½ tbsp. Italian seasoning
- ¼ tbsp. black pepper
- 1 cup reduced-fat shredded mozzarella cheese shredded
- ½ cup cucumber grated
- ½ cup plain non-fat Greek yogurt
- ½ tbsp. garlic cloves crushed

Directions:

1. Preheat the oven to 425°F. Bake the cauliflower "rice" until golden brown on a baking sheet lined with parchment paper. Allow to cool after removing from the oven (keep the oven on and save the parchment paper for later). Squeeze the cauliflower in a cheesecloth or kitchen towel to remove any extra liquid.
2. Incorporate the cauliflower, eggs, parmesan cheese, and ¼ teaspoon of salt in a large mixing basin; whisk to combine.
3. Place the cauliflower mixture on a parchment-lined baking sheet and form it into a 12-inch pizza-shaped circle.
4. Toss the chicken strips, olives, Italian seasoning, and pepper together in a medium mixing basin.
5. On top of the cauliflower crust, arrange chicken pieces (cut into very fine strips) and olives, then top with mozzarella cheese. Preheat oven to 425°F and bake for 20 minutes, or until golden brown.
6. Make the tzatziki sauce while the cauliflower pizza dough is baking. Combine the cucumbers, yogurt, garlic, and ¼ teaspoon of salt in a mixing bowl (optional).
7. Cut the cauliflower pizza into four wedges and serve with tzatziki on the side.

Nutrition: Calories: 422 kcal; Carbs: 33 g; Protein: 4 g; Fat: 6 g; Saturated Fat: 25gFiber: 1 g; Sugar: 6 g.

50. 2-Ingredient Peanut Butter Energy Bites

Servings: 1
Difficulty: 2
Preparation Time: 5 minutes
Cooking Time: 0 minutes
Optavia Counts: 0 lean/ 0 green/ 1 healthy fat/ 1 condiments
Ingredients:

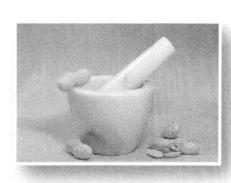

- Bar Optavia essential creamy double peanut butter crisp bar
- 1 tbsp. powdered peanut butter
- 1 tbsp. water

Directions:

1. In a small bowl, combine the powdered peanut butter with water to make a smooth paste.
2. Microwave the Creamy Double Peanut Butter Crisp Bar for 15 seconds or until soft on a microwave-safe dish.
3. To make a dough, combine the heated bits of the bar with the peanut butter.
4. Form four bite-sized balls using a cookie scoop or your finger. Place in the refrigerator until ready to eat.

Nutrition: Calories: 235 kcal; Carbs: 39 g; Protein: 4 g; Fat: 6 g; Saturated Fat: 25gFiber: 1 g; Sugar: 6 g.

51. Thin Mint Cookies

Servings: 1
Difficulty: 2
Preparation Time: 10 minutes
Cooking Time: 16 minutes
Optavia Counts: 1 lean/ 0 green/ 2 healthy fat/ 1 condiments
Ingredients:

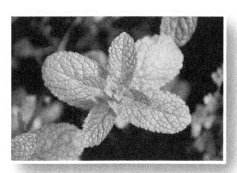

- 2 sachet Optavia essential decadent double chocolate brownie
- 2 bar Optavia essential chocolate mint cookie crisp bars
- 1 tbsp. liquid egg substitute
- 2 tbsp. unsweetened almond milk (optional)
- 2 tbsp. cashew milk (optional)
- ¼ tbsp. mint extract

Directions:

1. Preheat the oven to 350°F.
2. Soften Chocolate Mint Cookie Crisp Bars in the microwave for 15 to 20 seconds.
3. Combine the Decadent Double Chocolate Brownies, liquid egg substitute, milk (unsweetened almond or cashew), and mint essence in a small mixing bowl. Microwave crunch bars should be added at this point (will break apart into tiny pieces).
4. On a parchment-lined baking sheet, form the batter into eight cookie-shaped pieces.
5. Preheat oven to 350°F and bake for 12 to 15 minutes, or until firm.

Nutrition: Calories: 235 kcal; Carbs: 28 g; Protein: 4 g; Fat: 6 g; Saturated Fat: 25 g; Fiber: 1 g; Sugar: 4.9 g.

52. Red Velvet Whoopie Pies

Servings: 1
Difficulty: 2
Preparation Time: 10 minutes
Cooking Time: 20 minutes
Optavia Counts: 1 lean/ 0 green/ 3 healthy fat/ 6 condiments
Ingredients:

- 2 sachet Optavia essential golden chip pancakes
- 2 sachet Optavia essential chewy chocolate chip cookie
- ½ tbsp. unsweetened cocoa powder (optional)
- ½ tbsp. baking powder
- ½ cup unsweetened vanilla almond milk (optional)
- ½ cup cashew milk (optional)
- 6 tbsp. liquid egg substitute
- 1 tbsp. apple cider vinegar
- Dash red food coloring (optional)
- 1 can cooking spray
- ½ cup low-fat cream cheese
- 1-2 packet zero-calorie sugar substitute

Directions:

1. Preheat the oven to 350°F. In a medium-sized mixing bowl, combine Golden Pancakes, Chewy Chocolate Chip Cookies, cocoa powder, and baking powder. Mix in the milk, egg, and apple cider vinegar until a batter-like consistency is achieved. Add a smidgeon of red food coloring if desired.
2. Divide the mixture evenly among eight slots in a normal or heart-shaped muffin pan previously gently oiled (only fill a third of each tin slot). Cook for 15–20 minutes, or until a toothpick inserted in the center comes out clean. Combine the cream cheese and sugar substitute (to taste) while the muffins are baking. After the muffins have cooled, cut them in half horizontally, 1 tablespoon of cream cheese filling on the bottom half of each muffin, followed by the remaining muffin halves.

Nutrition: Calories: 104.6 kcal; Carbs: 28 g; Protein: 4 g; Fat: 6 g; Saturated Fat: 25 g; Fiber: 1 g; Sugar: 4 g.

53. Mint Chocolate Cheesecake Muffins

Servings: 1
Difficulty: 2
Preparation Time: 10 minutes
Cooking Time: 0 minutes
Optavia Counts: 0 lean/ 1 green/ 1 healthy fat/ 2 condiments
Ingredients:

- 4 sachet essential chocolate mint cookie crisp bars
- 12 oz. low-fat Greek yogurt
- 2 tbsp. sugar-free chocolate pudding mix
- ¼ tbsp. peppermint extract
- 8 small fresh mint leaves (optional)

Directions:

1. Eight cupcake liners should be lined in a standard-sized muffin pan. Each Chocolate Mint Cookie Crisp Bar should be cut in two. Microwave the bar halves crunch-side down on a microwave-safe dish for 20 to 30 seconds, or until softened. Press down each piece into the bottom of a cupcake liner to make a thin crust. Continue until all of the cupcake liners have been filled. Combine low-fat plain Greek yogurt and sugar-free, fat-free chocolate pudding mix in a large mixing bowl until well mixed.
2. Divide the yogurt and pudding mixture evenly among the muffin liners. Freeze for 30-60 minutes, or until completely solid. If preferred, garnish with fresh mint leaves and serve right away.

Nutrition: Calories: 291 kcal; Carbs: 36 g; Protein: 4 g; Fat: 6 g; Saturated Fat: 25 g; Fiber: 1 g; Sugar: 9 g.

54. Neapolitan Froyo Popsicles

Servings: 1
Difficulty: 2
Preparation Time: 25 minutes
Cooking Time: 0 minutes
Optavia Counts: 0 lean/ 0 green/ 6 healthy fat/ 1 condiment
Ingredients:

- 1 cup unsweetened vanilla almond milk divided (optional)
- 1 cup cashew milk divided (optional)
- 1 cup low-fat Greek yogurt divided
- 1 sachet Octavia essentials creamy chocolate shake
- 1 sachet Optavia essential creamy vanilla shake
- 1 sachet Optavia essential wild strawberry shake
- 1 packet zero-calorie sugar substitute

Directions:

1. In a blender, combine ⅓ cup milk (unsweetened vanilla almond or cashew), ⅔ cup plain Greek yogurt, Creamy Chocolate Shake, and ⅓ of a packet of sugar replacement; mix until smooth.
2. Place the mixture in the freezer for 15 minutes after equally distributing it across the bottoms of 6 big popsicle molds (to help set the popsicles a bit).
3. Steps 1–2 are repeated with the Creamy Vanilla Shake (15 minutes in the freezer), and finally the Wild Strawberry Shake. Freeze for at least 4 hours or overnight after repeating all of the instructions.

Nutrition: Calories: 235 kcal; Carbs: 39 g; Protein: 4 g; Fat: 6 g; Saturated Fat: 25 g; Fiber: 1 g; Sugar: 6 g.

55. Pizza, Spaghetti and Marinara Sauce

Servings: 1
Difficulty: 2
Preparation Time: 5 minutes
Cooking Time: 3 minutes
Optavia Counts: 0 lean/ 0 green/ 1 healthy fat/ 8 condiment
Ingredients:

- ½ can (12-oz.) no salt added tomato paste
- ½ can (12-oz.) no salt added tomato sauce
- 2 tbsp. olive oil
- 1 tbsp. zero-calorie sugar substitute
- ½ tbsp. lemon juice
- 1 tbsp. Italian seasoning
- 1 tbsp. garlic powder
- 1 tbsp. onion powder
- ⅛ tbsp. pepper

Directions:

1. In a saucepan, combine all of the ingredients. Over medium heat, come to a boil. Reduce the heat to low and cook for 18-20 minutes.
2. Yields 2 cups.

Nutrition: Calories: 235 kcal; Carbs: 39 g; Protein: 4 g; Fat: 6 g; Saturated Fat: 25 g; Fiber: 1 g; Sugar: 6 g.

56. Cranberry Sweet Potato Muffins

Servings: 2
Difficulty: 3
Preparation Time: 5 minutes
Cooking Time: 25 minutes
Optavia Counts: 1 lean/ 2 green/ 2 healthy fat/ 5 condiment
Ingredients:

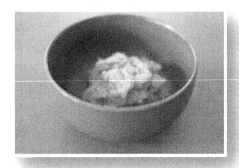

- ¾ cup cooked, mashed sweet potato
- 2 eggs
- 1 tbsp. vanilla extract
- ½ cup brown sugar (increase to ⅔ cup for a sweeter muffin)
- ⅔ cup milk (cow or plant-based)
- ¼ cup oil (I use avocado)
- 1 tbsp. cinnamon
- 1 tbsp. baking soda
- 1 ½ cups flour (I used white whole wheat)
- 1 cup fresh or frozen cranberries (or ⅓– ½ cup Craisins or chocolate chips)

Directions:

1. In a large mixing basin, combine sweet potato, eggs, vanilla, brown sugar, milk, oil, and cinnamon.
2. Stir in the flour and baking soda until barely mixed.
3. Add fresh cranberries or chocolate chips to the mix.
4. Scoop into muffin pans and bake for 20-22 minutes at 375 degrees, or until a toothpick inserted in the middle comes out clean.
5. Allow to cool fully before serving.

Nutrition: Calories: 296 kcal; Carbs: 43 g; Protein: 4 g; Fat: 6 g; Saturated Fat: 25 g; Fiber: 1 g; Sugar: 8 g.

57. Mini Peanut Butter Cups

Servings: 2
Difficulty: 2
Preparation Time: 0 minutes
Cooking Time: 15 minutes
Optavia Counts: 0 lean/ 0 green/ 3 healthy fat/ 0 condiment
Ingredients:

- Sachet optavia essential decadent double chocolate brownie
- 10 tbsp. unsweetened vanilla almond milk divided (optional)
- 10 tbsp. cashew milk divided (optional)
- ¼ cup powdered peanut butter

Directions:

1. Combine Decadent Double Chocolate Brownie and 6 tablespoons of almond milk (or cashew milk) in a small mixing bowl until smooth; leave aside. Combine powdered peanut butter with the remaining almond milk (or cashew milk) in a separate small dish until smooth and creamy, but not too thin.
2. Place the brownie and peanut butter mixes in separate resealable plastic bags, medium to large in size. To make piping bags, cut a little piece off one tip of each bag.
3. Fill the bottom third of 20 holes in a small round or heart-shaped silicone baking mold with brownie batter. In the center of each slot, pipe a little quantity of peanut butter on top of the brownie. Fill each hole with the remaining brownie batter, which should be piped on top of the peanut butter to cover it.
4. Freeze for at least 2 hours, or until firm.

Nutrition: Calories: 470 kcal; Carbs: 33 g; Protein: 4 g; Fat: 6 g; Saturated Fat: 25 g; Fiber: 7 g; Sugar: 5 g.

58. Skinny Chicken Queso

Servings: 2
Difficulty: 2
Preparation Time: 10 minutes
Cooking Time: 20 minutes
Optavia Counts: 1 lean/ 4 green/ 3 healthy fat/ 0 condiment
Ingredients:

- 12 oz. boneless skinless chicken breast shredded
- ½ cup reduced fat sharp cheddar cheese shredded
- ¾ cup low-fat Greek yogurt
- 4 tbsp. reduced-fat cream cheese
- 1 cup diced tomatoes w/ green chilies
- ½ cup fresh cilantro chopped
- 1 pound mini sweet peppers halved
- ½ cup celery halved

Directions:

1. Preheat the oven to 350°F.
2. Cook and shred the chicken, then combine it with the sharp cheddar cheese, softened cream cheese, and Greek plain yogurt in a mixing basin, stir well, and pour into a lightly oiled casserole dish.
3. Bake for 20 minutes, or until completely heated.
4. Chop the cilantro, tiny sweet peppers (halved lengthwise, stems and seeds removed), and celery into half for dipping while the cheese is cooking.
5. Serve immediately.

Nutrition: Calories: 419 kcal; Carbs: 33 g; Protein: 4 g; Fat: 6 g; Saturated Fat: 25 g; Fiber: 1 g; Sugar: 8.2 g.

59. Personal Biscuit Pizza

Servings: 2
Difficulty: 2
Preparation Time: 5 minutes
Cooking Time: 15 minutes
Optavia Counts: 0 lean/ 0 green/ 2 healthy fat/ 2 condiment
Ingredients:

- Sachet Optavia select buttermilk cheddar herb biscuit
- 1 tbsp. cold water
- 1 can cooking spray
- 1 tbsp. Rao's Homemade sauce
- ¼ cup reduced-fat cheese

Directions:

1. Preheat the oven to 350°F.
2. Combine the biscuit mix and water in a tiny, thin, circular crust shape on a foil-lined baking sheet lightly coated with cooking spray. Cook for 10 minutes in the oven
3. After baking for 10 minutes, cover with tomato sauce (such as Rao's Homemade) and mozzarella, and bake for another 4-5 minutes, or until the cheese is melted.

Nutrition: Calories: 235 kcal; Carbs: 39 g; Protein: 4 g; Fat: 6 g; Saturated Fat: 25 g; Fiber: 1 g; Sugar: 6 g.

60. Mini Cranberry Orange Spiced Cheesecake

Servings: 2
Difficulty: 1
Preparation Time: 5 minutes
Cooking Time: 15 minutes
Optavia Counts: 0 lean/ 0 green/ 1 healthy fat/ 2 condiment
Ingredients:

- Sachet Optavia Honey Chili Cranberry Nut Bars
- 1 ½ cups low-fat Greek yogurt
- 1 tbsp. sugar-free cheesecake pudding
- 1 tbsp. orange zest

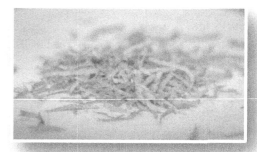

Directions:

1. Using 8 cupcake liners, line a standard-sized muffin pan.
2. Each Honey Chili Cranberry Nut Bar should be cut in half. Microwave the bar halves crunch-side down on a microwave-safe dish for 20 to 30 seconds, or until softened.

Nutrition: Calories: 235 kcal; Carbs: 39 g; Protein: 4 g; Fat: 6 g; Saturated Fat: 25 g; Fiber: 1 g; Sugar: 6 g.

61. Caprese Pizza Bites

Servings: 2
Difficulty: 3
Preparation Time: 12 minutes
Cooking Time: 10 minutes
Optavia Counts: 0 lean/ 3 green/ 3 healthy fat/ 2 condiment
Ingredients:

- Sachet Optavia Buttermilk Cheddar Herb Biscuit
- ½ cup unsweetened almond milk
- 1 tbsp. olive oil
- 1 can cooking spray
- 1 cup basil leaves
- 8 oz fresh mozzarella log chopped
- 4 small Roma tomatoes sliced
- 1 tbsp. balsamic vinegar

Directions:

1. Preheat the oven to 450°F.
2. Combine the Buttermilk Cheddar Herb Biscuit, milk (unsweetened almond or cashew milk), and oil in a medium-sized mixing dish.
3. In a standard-sized, lightly-greased muffin pan, divide the biscuit mixture evenly among the 12 holes.
4. Each muffin pan slot should be layered with a slice of mozzarella, a slice of tomato, and a few basil leaves.
5. Bake for 10 to 12 minutes, or until the biscuit mixture is golden brown and the cheese has melted.
6. Before serving, drizzle the tops with balsamic vinegar.

Nutrition: Calories: 205 kcal; Carbs: 31 g; Protein: 4 g; Fat: 6 g; Saturated Fat: 25 g; Fiber: 1 g; Sugar: 7 g.

62. Silky Peanut Butter Cookies

Servings: 3
Difficulty: 1
Preparation Time: 10 minutes
Cooking Time: 15 minutes
Optavia Counts: 0 lean/ 0 green/ 1 healthy fat/ 6 condiment
Ingredients:

- Sachet Optavia essential silky peanut butter shake
- ¼ tbsp. baking powder
- ¼ tbsp. unsweetened original (optional)
- 1 tbsp. butter (optional)
- ¼ tbsp. vanilla extract
- 1 can light cooking spray
- ⅛ tbsp. sea salt (optional)

Directions:

1. Preheat the oven to 350°F. Spray a baking pan with cooking spray and line it with foil.
2. Combine the first two ingredients in a medium-sized mixing basin. Stir in the milk (¼ cup unsweetened original vanilla almond or cashew milk), butter (melted or softened), and vanilla essence until everything is thoroughly mixed (it will appear dry, but continue mixing until a dough forms; add another tablespoon of milk if necessary)
3. Scoop the dough into 8 tiny balls using a small cookie scoop and place on a foil-lined, lightly oiled baking sheet. Flatten the mounds with a fork to make a crisscross design. Season with salt on the tops (optional).
4. Bake for 10 to 12 minutes, or until the sides are gently browned. If preferred, serve with unsweetened original or vanilla almond milk (optional).

Nutrition: Calories: 119 kcal; Carbs: 27 g; Protein: 4 g; Fat: 6 g; Saturated Fat: 25 g; Fiber: 1 g; Sugar: 8 g.

63. Smash Potato Grilled Cheese

Servings: 3
Difficulty: 2
Preparation Time: 10 minutes
Cooking Time: 25 minutes
Optavia Counts: 0 lean/ 1 green/ 1 healthy fat/ 0 condiment
Ingredients:

- Sachet Optavia Essential Smashed Potatoes
- 1 cup water
- 1 cup Reduced-Fat Cheddar Cheese shredded (optional)*

Directions:

1. A waffle iron should be preheated.
2. Mix Optavia Essential Smashed Potatoes and water in a medium microwave-safe bowl until fully mixed. Microwave for 1 ½ minutes on High, then stir.
3. Coat a heated waffle iron lightly with cooking spray before pouring the batter into it. Close the cover and cook for 10 to 12 minutes, or until done.
4. Open the cover and spread half of the waffle with cheese of your choice (low-fat shredded Cheddar, mozzarella, or Pepper Jack) (two of the four). Fold the second half of the waffle over, shut the waffle iron top, and cook for another 1 to 2 minutes, or until the cheese has melted.

Nutrition: Calories: 302 kcal; Carbs: 39 g; Protein: 4 g; Fat: 6 g; Saturated Fat: 25 g; Fiber: 1 g; Sugar: 9 g.

64. Buffalo Cauliflower Wings

Servings: 3
Difficulty: 2
Preparation Time: 5 minutes
Cooking Time: 30 minutes
Optavia Counts: 0 lean/ 1 green/ 3 healthy fat/ 3 condiment
Ingredients:

- Sachet optavia buttermilk cheddar herb biscuit
- ½ cup water
- 1 cup cauliflower florets
- 1 can cooking spray
- ¼ cup hot buffalo sauce
- ½ tbsp. unsalted butter melted
- ¼ cup low-fat Greek yogurt
- 1 tbsp. dry ranch dressing mix

Directions:

1. Preheat the oven to 425°F.
2. Combine buttermilk cheddar herb biscuits and water in a medium-sized mixing dish. Toss the cauliflower florets in the batter until they are uniformly covered.
3. Place cauliflower florets on a gently oiled foil-lined baking sheet. Preheat oven to 350°F and bake for 20 minutes. Combine the spicy sauce and butter in a separate bowl. Toss in the roasted cauliflower florets to coat them. Return to the baking sheet and bake for 7 to 10 minutes more.
4. Combine yogurt and ranch dressing mix in a small bowl. With the ranch dip, serve the cauliflower wings.

Nutrition: Calories: 174 kcal; Carbs: 28 g; Protein: 4 g; Fat: 6 g; Saturated Fat: 25 g; Fiber: 1 g; Sugar: 6 g.

65. Cheddar & Chive Savory Smashed Potato Waffles

Servings: 3
Difficulty: 2
Preparation Time: 7 minutes
Cooking Time: 15 minutes
Optavia Counts: 2 lean/ 2 green/ 3 healthy fat/ 1 condiment
Ingredients:

- Sachet optavia essential roasted garlic creamy smashed potatoes
- ½ cup unsweetened almond milk
- ½ cup reduced-fat cheddar cheese shredded
- ½ cup liquid egg substitute
- 2 medium turkey bacon chopped
- ¼ cup scallions chopped
- 1 can cooking spray
- ¼ cup low-fat Greek yogurt

Directions:

1 Mix Garlic Creamy Smashed Potatoes, milk, cheese, and egg replacement in a medium-sized mixing basin until fully blended. Cook 1 to 2 slices turkey bacon as directed on the package, and chop into tiny pieces Add the scallions, chopped. Gently fold all of the ingredients together.
2 Pour the batter onto a waffle iron lightly oiled and heated. Bake for 5 to 7 minutes, or until golden brown, with the lid closed. Remove waffle from waffle iron with care and serve.

Nutrition: Calories: 262 kcal; Carbs: 43 g; Protein: 4 g; Fat: 6 g; Saturated Fat: 25 g; Fiber: 1 g; Sugar: 9.3 g.

66. Very Veggie Dip

Servings: 3
Difficulty: 1
Preparation Time: 15 minutes
Cooking Time: 0 minutes
Optavia Counts: 0 lean/ 3 green/ 2 healthy fat/ 4 condiment
Ingredients:

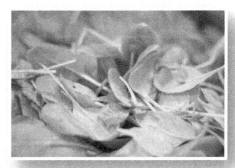

- 1 cup spinach
- 1 cup broccoli (optional)
- 1 ½ tbsp. light sour cream
- 1 tbsp. light mayonnaise
- 1 tbsp. scallions chopped
- 1 tbsp. lemon juice
- ¼ tbsp. chili powder
- ⅛ tbsp. cayenne pepper (optional)
- 1 pinch fresh nutmeg (optional)

Directions:

1 Whirl (mix) all of the ingredients in a tiny mini chopper or food processor. If you don't have a processor, finely chop everything and mix it together.
2 Serve with a side of vegetables. You'll need 2 greens worth of various vegetables. This recipe serves 3 people.

Nutrition: Calories: 235 kcal; Carbs: 39 g; Protein: 4 g; Fat: 6 g; Saturated Fat: 25 g; Fiber: 1 g; Sugar: 6 g.

67. Pinto's & Cheese Fueling Hack

Servings: 3
Difficulty: 1
Preparation Time: 3 minutes
Cooking Time: 1minute
Optavia Counts: 0 lean/ 1 green/ 1 healthy fat/ 3 condiment
Ingredients:

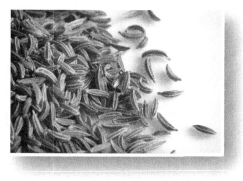

- Sachet Optavia sour cream & chives smashed potatoes
- ⅛ tbsp. cayenne pepper
- 1 tbsp. cumin
- 1 tbsp. reduced-fat cheddar cheese shredded
- 1 tbsp. cholula hot sauce

Directions:

1. Prepare the Optavia Sour Cream & Chives Smashed Potatoes according to the package directions.
2. Mix in the cumin and cayenne pepper well.
3. Enjoy with Cholula and reduced-fat cheddar cheese.

Nutrition: Calories: 421 kcal; Carbs: 32 g; Protein: 4 g; Fat: 6 g; Saturated Fat: 25 g; Fiber: 1 g; Sugar: 4 g.

68. Personal Portobello Mushroom Pizzas

Servings: 4
Difficulty: 2
Preparation Time: 11 minutes
Cooking Time: 5 minutes
Optavia Counts: 0 lean/ 1 green/ 1 healthy fat/ 3 condiment
Ingredients:

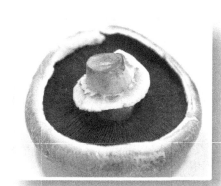

- 1 can light cooking spray
- 2 (2-oz.) medium Portobello mushroom caps
- ¼ cup no sugar added Italian tomato sauce
- 4 oz. reduced-fat mozzarella cheese
- 1 tbsp. fresh basil shredded (optional)

Directions:

1. Preheat the oven to broil.
2. Place the mushroom caps on a gently oiled foil-lined baking sheet. Coat the tops with cooking spray. Cook for 3 to 4 minutes on each side under the broiler until tender.
3. Spread the tomato sauce evenly across each cap, then top with the cheese and basil. Broil for another 2 to 3 minutes, or until the cheese is completely melted.

Nutrition: Calories: 235 kcal; Carbs: 39 g; Protein: 4 g; Fat: 6 g; Saturated Fat: 25 g; Fiber: 1 g; Sugar: 6 g.

69. Grilled Mahi with Jicama Slaw

Servings: 4
Difficulty: 2
Preparation Time: 20 minutes
Cooking Time: 10 minutes
Optavia Counts: 1 lean/ 3 green/ 1 healthy fat/ 3 condiment
Ingredients:

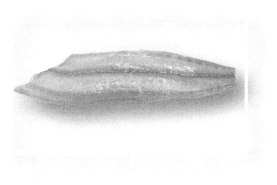

- 2 tbsp. lime juice divided
- 1 tbsp. salt divided
- 1 tbsp. black pepper divided
- 4 (8oz.) medium mahi-mahi fillets
- 2 tbsp. extra-virgin olive oil divided
- 1 cup jicama sliced
- 1 cup cucumber sliced
- 1 cup watercress chopped
- 1 cup alfalfa sprouts

Directions:

1. In a small bowl, combine 1 teaspoon of lime juice, ½ teaspoon each of salt and pepper, and 2 tablespoons of oil. Brush the olive oil mixture evenly over the mahi-mahi fillets.
2. Grill the mahi-mahi (8 oz.) for 5 minutes on each side (internal temperature of 145°F) over medium-high heat until done.
3. Jicama (thinly cut into long strips like matchsticks), cucumber (thinly cut into long strips like matchsticks), watercress, and alfalfa sprouts are combined in a dish for the slaw. In a small bowl, combine 2 teaspoons of lime juice, ½ teaspoon of salt and pepper, and 2 tablespoons of extra virgin olive oil. Drizzle the dressing over the slaw and toss to mix.

Nutrition: Calories: 209 kcal; Carbs: 26 g; Protein: 4 g; Fat: 6 g; Saturated Fat: 25 g; Fiber: 1 g; Sugar: 5.8 g.

70. Taco Stuffed Portobellos

Servings: 4
Difficulty: 2
Preparation Time: 10 minutes
Cooking Time: 15 minutes
Optavia Counts: 1 lean/ 1 green/ 1 healthy fat/ 9 condiments
Ingredients:

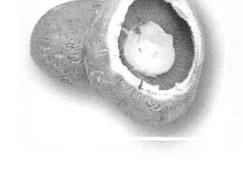

- 4 large portobello mushroom caps
- 1 pound lean ground beef
- 2 tbsp. onion chopped
- ¼ cup poblano peppers diced
- 1 small garlic clove minced
- 1 (14 ½ oz.) can diced tomatoes
- 1 tbsp. cumin
- 1 tbsp. chili powder
- ½ tbsp. dried parsley
- ¼ tbsp. salt (optional)
- ¼ tbsp. black pepper
- 4 oz reduced-fat cheddar cheese spiraled

Directions:

1. Preheat the broiler to a Low setting. Remove the stems and scrape the gills off the underside of the mushroom cap, discarding them. Place the mushrooms on a baking pan and brush with olive oil. Broil for 4 to 5 minutes, or until tender.
2. Meanwhile, sear the beef in a large pan with the onion, pepper, and garlic over medium-high heat. Reduce the heat to Low, add the tomatoes and seasonings, and continue to cook for 10 minutes.
3. Scoop one piece of the mixture into each mushroom cap after dividing the mixture into four portions (serve any excess filling alongside the mushroom). On top of each mushroom, sprinkle around 1 oz. of cheese.

Nutrition: Calories: 317 kcal; Carbs: 43 g; Protein: 4 g; Fat: 6 g; Saturated Fat: 25 g; Fiber: 1 g; Sugar: 7.2 g.

71. Mini Pepper Nachos

Servings: 4
Difficulty: 2
Preparation Time: 5 minutes
Cooking Time: 15 minutes
Optavia Counts: 1 lean/ 2 green/ 3 healthy fat/ 4 condiments
Ingredients:

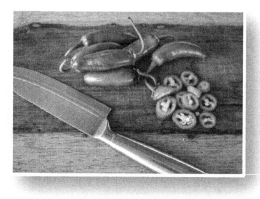

- ¼ cup jalapeno peppers diced
- 1 (12-oz.) can canned chicken breast drained
- 6 oz. avocado mashed
- ½ cup plain non-fat Greek yogurt
- 2 cups reduced-fat cheddar cheese shredded
- 1 tbsp. chili powder
- 24 small mini bell peppers halved
- ¼ cup scallions chopped
- 4 dash light cooking spray
- ½ cup salsa (optional)

Directions:

1. In a lightly oiled pan, cook the diced jalapeño until tender.
2. In a medium mixing bowl, combine the jalapeño, chicken, avocado, yogurt, one cup of cheese, and chili powder.
3. In a large casserole dish, arrange the tiny bell peppers in a single layer. Fill with chicken mixture, top with remaining cheese, and broil for 2-4 minutes, or until cheese has melted.
4. If preferred, garnish with scallions and serve with salsa.

Nutrition: Calories: 309 kcal; Carbs: 20 g; Protein: 4 g; Fat: 6 g; Saturated Fat: 25 g; Fiber: 1 g; Sugar: 8.1 g.

72. Curried Chicken Salad Wraps

Servings: 4
Difficulty: 1
Preparation Time: 5 minutes
Cooking Time: 3 minutes
Optavia Counts: 1 lean/ 3 green/ 2 healthy fat/ 3 condiments
Ingredients

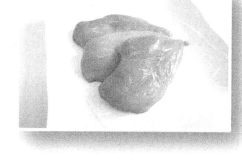

- 10 oz. canned chicken breast
- ½ cup plain non-fat Greek yogurt
- ½ cup celery diced
- 2 tbsp. curry powder
- 2 tbsp. fresh parsley chopped
- ¼ tbsp. salt
- ¼ tbsp. black pepper
- 1 large Romaine lettuce
- ⅔ oz. peanuts chopped

Directions:

1. In a medium mixing dish, combine the chicken, yogurt, celery, herbs, and spices.
2. To make the wraps, spread chicken salad on lettuce leaves, sprinkle with peanuts and roll them up.

Nutrition: Calories: 167 kcal; Carbs: 21 g; Protein: 4 g; Fat: 6 g; Saturated Fat: 25 g; Fiber: 1 g; Sugar: 4.3 g.

73. Cilantro Lime Fish

Servings: 4
Difficulty: 1
Preparation Time: 10 minutes
Cooking Time: 20 minutes
Optavia Counts: 1 lean/ 0 green/ 1 healthy fat/ 4 condiments
Ingredients:

- 2 pounds white fish fillets
- ⅓ cup lime juice
- 1 tbsp. dried cilantro
- 1 tbsp. olive oil
- ¼ tbsp. red pepper flakes (optional)
- Salt/pepper to taste

Directions:

1. Preheat the oven to 350°F.
2. In a 13X9 baking dish, place the fish. Season to taste with salt and pepper. Combine the remaining ingredients in a small bowl. Pour the sauce over the fish. Cook for 15-20 minutes at 350°F.

Nutrition: Calories: 295 kcal; Carbs: 6.9 g; Protein: 4 g; Fat: 6 g; Saturated Fat: 25 g; Fiber: 1 g; Sugar: 7 g.

74. West Indies Shrimp

Servings: 4
Difficulty: 3
Preparation Time: 10 minutes
Cooking Time: 15 minutes
Optavia Counts: 1 lean/ 1 green/ 1 healthy fat/ 5 condiments
Ingredients:

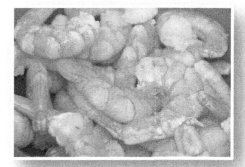

- 12 cups water
- 2 pounds unpeeled medium shrimp
- 2 tsp. Old Bay seasoning
- 1 cup chopped onion
- 1 cup chopped green bell pepper
- ⅔ cup cider vinegar
- 1 ½ tbsp. vegetable oil
- 1 tsp. salt
- ¼ tsp. black pepper

Directions:

1. In a big saucepan, bring water to a boil. Cook for 3 minutes, or until shrimp is cooked through. Drain and set aside to cool fully. Fill a big zip-top plastic bag halfway with shrimp. Seal the bag and marinate in the refrigerator for 30 minutes, rotating it occasionally. Remove the shrimp from the bag and set aside the marinade. Peel the shrimp and throw them in a large mixing basin. Toss in the remaining marinade, gently tossing to coat.

Nutrition: Calories: 57 kcal; Carbs: 39 g; Protein: 4 g; Fat: 1.8 g; Saturated Fat: 25 g; Fiber: 1 g; Sugar: 2 g.

CHAPTER 6.

DINNER RECIPES

75. Air Fryer Asparagus

Serving: 1
Difficulty: 1
Preparation Time: 5 minutes
Cooking Time: 8 minutes
Optavia Counts: 0 lean/ 1 green/ 0 healthy fat/ 2 condiments
Ingredients:

- Nutritional yeast
- Olive oil non-stick spray
- 1 bunch of asparagus

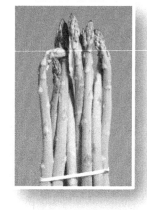

Directions:
1. Wash the asparagus. Do not forget to trim off thick, woody ends.
2. Coat with olive oil spray and sprinkle with yeast.
3. In your Instant Crisp Air Fryer, lay the asparagus in a single layer. Set the temperature to 360°F. Limit the time to eight minutes.

Nutrition: Calories: 17; Fat: 4 g; Protein: 9 g.

76. Avocado Fries

Serving: 1
Difficulty: 1
Preparation Time: 10 minutes
Cooking Time: 7 minutes
Optavia Counts: 0 lean/ 0 green/ 0 healthy fat/ 3 condiments
Ingredients:

- 1 Avocado
- ⅛ tsp. salt
- ¼ cup of panko breadcrumbs
- Bean liquid (aquafaba) from a 15-ounce can of white or garbanzo beans

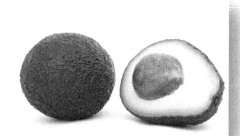

Directions:
1. Peel, pit, and slice up avocado.
2. Toss salt and breadcrumbs together in a bowl. Place the aquafaba into another bowl.
3. Dredge slices of avocado first in the aquafaba and then in panko, making sure you are evenly coating.
4. Place coated avocado slices into a single layer in the Instant Crisp Air Fryer. Set temperature to 390°F and time to 5 minutes.
5. Serve with your favorite Keto dipping sauce!

Nutrition: Calories: 102; Fat: 22 g; Protein: 9 g; Sugar: 1 g.

77. Cheesy Zucchini

Serving: 1
Difficulty: 1
Preparation Time: 5 minutes
Cooking Time: 15 minutes
Optavia Counts: 1 lean/ 1 green/ 3 healthy fat/ 3 condiments
Ingredients:

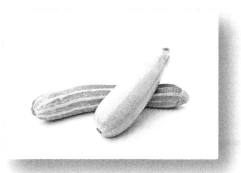

- ¼ pound zucchini
- ¼ tsp. sea salt
- 1/16 cups grated parmesan cheese
- 1/16 cups flour
- ½ cloves garlic
- ½ tbsp. extra virgin olive oil
- ¼ large egg
- Black pepper

Directions:

1. Put the grated zucchini into a colander over the sink. Add your salt and toss it to mix properly, then leave it to settle for about 10 minutes. Next, use a clean cheesecloth to drain the zucchini completely.
2. Combine drained zucchini, parmesan, garlic, flour, and the beaten egg in a large bowl, mix, and season with pepper and salt. Then, pour the olive oil into a skillet applying medium-high heat.
3. Use a tablespoon to scoop batter for each fritter. Put in the oil, and flatten using a spatula.
4. Allow cooking until the underside is richly golden brown; then flip over to the other side and cook.
5. Your delicious fried zucchini is ready to be served.

Nutrition: Calories: 163.1 kcal; Protein: 7.4 g; Fat: 8.8 g; Carbs: 18.0 g.

78. Veggie Crusty Pizza

Serving: 1
Difficulty: 3
Preparation Time: 15 minutes
Cooking Time: 30 minutes
Optavia Counts: 1 lean/ 2 green/ 2 healthy fat/ 2 condiments
Ingredients:

- ¼ cauliflower
- 1/16 parmesan cheese
- ½ egg
- ½ tsp. Italian seasoning
- 1/16 tsp. sea salt
- 1 cup mozzarella cheese
- ¼ cup spicy pizza sauce - Basil leaves

Directions:

1. Start by preheating the oven while lining the baking sheet with parchment paper. Cut the cauliflower into smaller portions. Grate the parmesan cheese and mozzarella.
2. Process the cauliflower into a fine powder and then place it in a bowl before putting it in the microwave. Let it soften for about 5-6 minutes. Transfer the microwaved cauliflower to a clean and dry kitchen towel. Allow it to cool. Once cooled, use the kitchen towel to wrap the cauliflower and then get rid of all the moisture by wringing out the towel. Keep squeezing it until all the water is gone.
3. Add in the cauliflower, Italian seasonings, parmesan cheese, egg, salt and mozzarella (1 cup).
4. Stir very well until everything is well combined. Transfer the combined mixture to the beforehand prepared baking sheet and press into a 10-inch round pan. Wait to bake until it turns a golden color.
5. Remove the baked crust from the oven and top with the spicy pizza sauce and mozzarella (the remaining 1 cup). Put it back in the oven for another 10 minutes, until the cheese melts and looks bubbly. Garnish with fresh basil leaves. You can also enjoy this with salad.

Nutrition: Calories: 508.2 kcal; Protein: 33.8 g; Fat: 32.7 g; Carbs: 19.6 g.

79. Tarragon Cauliflower

Serving: 1
Difficulty: 1
Preparation Time: 10 minutes
Cooking Time: 10 - 15 minutes
Optavia Counts: 0 lean/ 1 green/ 0 healthy fat/ 7 condiments
Ingredients:

- 2 cups cauliflower
- 1 tsp. sugar substitute
- ½ tbsp. chives
- 1 tbsp. lemon juice
- 1 tbsp. balsamic vinegar
- 1 tsp. tarragon
- 1 garlic clove
- Salt/pepper to taste

Directions:

1. Steam cauliflower until fork tender. Mince garlic. Squeeze the juice from the lemon.
2. Mix vinegar, dried chives, dried tarragon, sugar substitute, garlic, lemon juice.
3. Pour over hot cauliflower. Add salt and pepper. Blend mixture.

Nutrition: Calories: 64 kcal; Protein: 5 g; Fat: 1.2 g; Carbs: 12.6 g.

80. Winter Salad

Serving: 1
Difficulty: 1
Prep Time: 10 minutes
Cook Time: 10 – 15 minutes
Optavia Counts: 0 lean/ 4 green/ 1 healthy fat/ 4 condiments
Ingredients:

- 1 cup broccoli
- 1 cup cauliflower
- 1 cup cherry tomatoes
- ¼ cup olives
- 1 ½ tbsp. lemon juice
- ¼ tsp. garlic powder
- 1 tbsp. oil, preferably olive
- ¼ tsp. oregano
- ¼ tsp. salt

Directions:

1. Steam broccoli and cauliflower together until fork tender.
2. Blend lemon, oil, garlic, oregano and salt in a bowl.
3. Pour over the veggies.
4. Half the cherry tomatoes.
5. Slice the olives.
6. Stir in tomatoes and olives.

Nutrition: Calories: 99 kcal; Protein: 7.4 g; Fat: 0.6 g; Carbs: 19.9 g.

81. Energizing Mocha Smoothie

Serving: 1
Difficulty: 1
Preparation Time: 5 minutes
Cooking Time: 0 minutes
Optavia Counts: 1 lean/ 0 green/ 1 healthy fat/ 1 condiments
Ingredients:

- 1 Banana (frozen preferable)
- 1 tbsp. peanut butter
- 1 tbsp. cocoa powder
- ¼ cup Plain Yogurt
- ⅓ cup Brewed Coffee (preferable chilled)

Directions:

1. Place all ingredients in a food blender in the order listed and pulse until smooth, 1 to 2 minutes.
2. Divide the smoothie between two glasses and then serve it.

Nutrition: Calories: 117.1 kcal; Protein: 1.01 g; Fat: 3.6 g; Carbs: 20.1 g.

82. Flavored Sandwich Filling

Serving: 2
Difficulty: 1
Preparation Time: 5 minutes
Cooking Time: 0 minutes
Optavia Counts: 0 lean/ 6 green/ 1 healthy fat/ 1 condiment
Ingredients:

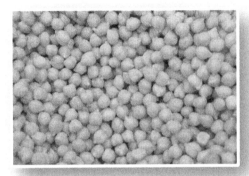

- 1 handful of chickpeas
- 1 soft baguette
- 8 to 10 olives (preferable black)
- 1 red onion
- 3 tbsp. vegan mayo
- ¼ English cucumber
- 1 radish
- 6 to 8 basil leaves (fresh preferable)
- Salt
- Black pepper

Directions:

1. Trim the green beans.
2. Slice in half 1 soft baguette.
3. Pit and slice the black olives in half.
4. Slice thinly the rinsed and dried onion.
5. Slice thinly the English cucumber and radish.
6. Grind the black pepper right before you mix it in the dish for an amazing flavor.
7. Take a medium bowl, add chickpeas in it, and then add the remaining ingredients.
8. Stir until well mixed and when ready, serve filling as a sandwich between two bread slices.

Nutrition: Calories: 356.7 kcal; Protein: 11.6 g; Fat: 7.5 g; Carbs: 60.6 g.

83. Angelic Pasta

Serving: 2
Difficulty: 1
Preparation Time: 10 minutes
Cooking Time: 10 minutes
Optavia Counts: 0 lean/ 1 green/ 2 healthy fat/ 4 condiment
Ingredients:

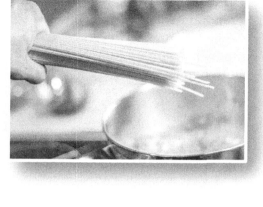

- 1 tbsp. olive oil
- 1 tsp. garlic
- 1 cup broccoli florets
- 1 cup pasta
- Pinch pepper flakes
- ⅛ cup shredded Parmesan cheese
- Salt
- Black Pepper

Directions:

1. Cut broccoli florets into small pieces, place in a heatproof bowl, cover with plastic wrap, then microwave for 3 to 5 minutes. Drain the broccoli well to remove all the moisture, then set aside until ready to use. Meanwhile, fill a medium saucepan halfway with water and set over medium-high heat. Bring the water to a boil, then add the pasta and spaghetti and cook until tender, 5 to 8 minutes.
2. Drain the pasta, return it to the pot, add the broccoli and cheese. Then stir in the salt, black pepper, and minced garlic until everything is well mixed

Nutrition: Calories: 353.1 kcal; Protein: 9.77 g; Fat: 10.1 g; Carbs: 34.30 g.

84. Free Tofu

Serving: 2
Difficulty: 1
Preparation Time: 35 minutes
Cooking Time: 8 minutes
Optavia Counts: 1 lean/ 1 green/ 3 healthy fat/ 8 condiment
Ingredients:

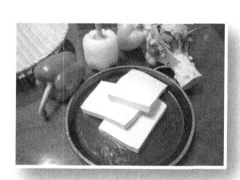

- ¾ pound firm tofu
- Vegetable oil
- Cornstarch
- 11 tbsp. butter
- 12 oz. small shallots
- 1-2 mild red chilies (preferable fresh)
- 12 garlic cloves
- 1 tbsp. ginger (preferable fresh)
- 1 tbsp. sweet soy sauce
- 1 tbsp. light soy sauce
- 1 tsp. dark soy sauce
- 1 tbsp. sugar
- 1 tbsp. black peppercorns
- 16 small and thin green onions

Directions:

1. Slice the shallots and red chills thinly. Mince the garlic cloves. Chop the ginger.
2. Use a mortar and pestle or a spice grinder to crush the black peppercorns coarsely.
3. Cut the green onions into 1 ¼" segments. Cut tofu into ¼-inch pieces. Place in a medium bowl, then add soy sauce and black pepper. Stir until tofu is coated, then let marinate for at least 30 minutes.
4. Next, take a medium frying pan, put it on medium-high heat, add oil, and when it is hot, add the tofu pieces and fry them for 2 to 3 minutes per side until they are golden brown and crispy.
5. When the tofu is done, garnish with sesame seeds and onions and then serve.

Nutrition: Calories: 154.3 kcal; Protein: 10.1 g; Fat: 11.3 g; Carbs: 3.8 g.

85. Unforgettable Mashed Potatoes

Serving: 2
Difficulty: 1
Preparation Time: 5 minutes
Cooking Time: 10 minutes
Optavia Counts: 1 lean/ 1 green/ 1 healthy fat/ 3 condiment
Ingredients:

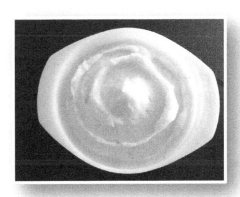

- 3 large russet potatoes
- 1 clove of garlic
- 1 cup of water
- 1 tbsp. white miso paste
- ⅓ cup almond milk (preferable unsweetened)

Extra:

- ⅓tsp. sea salt
- ¼ tsp. black pepper

Directions:

1. Peel the potatoes and cut them into ½ -inch rounds, then place them in a medium pot.
2. Cover potatoes with water, add 1 teaspoon of salt and garlic, place pot over medium-high heat and bring to a boil.
3. Turn the heat to medium and cook the potatoes for 10 to 15 minutes, until they are tender.
4. When they are done, drain the potatoes, return them to the pot and then add the milk and mash well until smooth.
5. Stir in remaining salt and black pepper, add miso paste and whip mixture with a hand blender until it reaches desired consistency.

Nutrition: Calories: 274.5 kcal; Protein: 5.5 g; Fat: 0.6 g; Carbs: 61.8 g.

86. Turkey Meatballs with Herbs

Serving: 2
Difficulty: 2
Preparation Time: 10-15 minutes
Cooking Time: 35 minutes
Optavia Counts: 1 lean/ 2 green/ 0 healthy fat/ 7 condiment
Ingredients:

- 19 oz. lean ground turkey
- 1 medium zucchini
- 15 oz. tomatoes with juice
- 1 tsp. garlic
- 1/2 medium onion
- 1 tsp. dried basil
- ½ tsp. red pepper flakes
- 1 tsp. dried oregano
- ¼ tsp. sea salt
- ¼ tsp. black pepper

Directions:

1. Preheat oven to 400°F. Peel and grate the zucchini into ⅓ cup.
2. Mince the garlic and the onions.
3. Blend all ingredients except tomatoes.
4. Create 18 golf ball-sized balls. Place the turkey balls in a baking dish.
5. Bake them for about 30 minutes.
6. Medium heat the skillet.
7. Add tomatoes with juices and meatballs.
8. Cook them for more than 5 minutes.

Nutrition: Calories: 316 kcal; Protein: 36 g; Fat: 15.5 g; Carbs: 10 g.

87. Zucchini Salmon Salad

Serving: 2
Difficulty: 1
Preparation Time: 5 minutes
Cooking Time: 10 minutes
Optavia Counts: 1 lean/ 1 green/ 1 healthy fat/ 4 condiment
Ingredients:

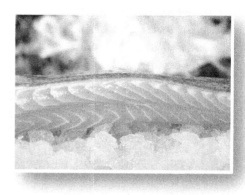

- 4 (150g each) salmon fillets
- 1 tbsp. soy sauce
- 3 zucchinis, sliced
- Salt and pepper to taste
- 1 tbsp. extra virgin olive oil
- 1 tbsp. sesame seeds
- Salt and pepper to taste

Directions:

1. Drizzle the salmon with soy sauce.
2. Heat a grill pan over a medium flame. Cook salmon on the grill on each side for 2–3 minutes.
3. Season the zucchini with salt and pepper and place it on the grill as well. Cook on each side until golden.
4. Place the zucchini, salmon, and the rest of the ingredients in a bowl.
5. Serve the salad fresh.

Nutrition: Calories: 224; Fat: 19 g; Protein: 18 g; Carbs: 0 g.

88. Pan Fried Salmon

Serving: 3
Difficulty: 2
 Preparation Time: 5 minutes
Cooking Time: 20 minutes
Optavia Counts: 1 lean/ 0 green/ 1 healthy fat/ 3 condiment
Ingredients:

- 2 x 150g salmon fillets
- Salt and pepper to taste
- 1 tsp. dried oregano
- 1 tsp. dried basil
- 1 tbsp. extra virgin olive oil

Directions:

1. Season the fish with salt, pepper, oregano, and basil.
2. Heat the oil in a pan and place the salmon in the hot oil, with the skin facing down.
3. Fry on each side for 2 minutes until golden brown and fragrant.
4. Serve the salmon warm and fresh.

Nutrition: Calories: 327 Fat: 25 g; Protein: 36 g; Carbs: 0.3 g.

89. Moussaka with Paprika

Serving: 3
Difficulty: 3
Preparation Time: 15 minutes
Cooking Time: 45 minutes
Optavia Counts: 1 lean/ 2 green/ 4 healthy fat/ 5 condiment
Ingredients:

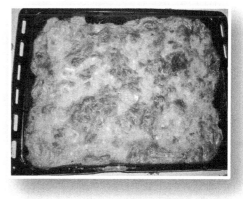

- 3 medium eggplant
- 1 cup ground chicken
- ⅓ cup white onion, diced
- 4 oz. Cheddar cheese
- 1 potato, sliced
- 1 tsp. olive oil
- 1 tsp. salt
- ½ cup milk
- 1 tbsp. butter
- 1 tbsp. ground paprika
- 1 tbsp. Italian seasoning
- 1 tsp. tomato paste

Directions:

1. Slice the eggplant lengthwise and sprinkle with salt. Chop the onion into small cubes. Pour olive oil into the pan and add the sliced potato. Fry the potato for 2 minutes on each side.
2. Then transfer it to the plate. Add the eggplant to the pan and fry it for 2 minutes on each side as well.
3. Pour milk into the pan and bring to a boil. Chop the cheddar cheese.
4. Add tomato paste, Italian seasoning, paprika, butter and cheddar cheese. Then mix the onion with the ground chicken. Arrange the sliced potatoes in a single layer in the casserole dish.
5. Then add ½ part of the sliced eggplant. Spread the eggplant with ½ part of the chicken mixture.
6. Then add the remaining eggplant. Pour the milk mixture over the eggplants.
7. Bake moussaka for 30 minutes at 355°F.

Nutrition: Calories: 387 kcal; Protein: 25.4 g; Fat: 21.2 g; Carbs: 26.3 g.

90. Tuna Salad

Serving: 3
Difficulty: 1
Preparation Time: 10 minutes
Cooking Time: 0
Optavia Counts: 1 lean/ 3 green/ 0 healthy fat/ 0 condiment
Ingredients:

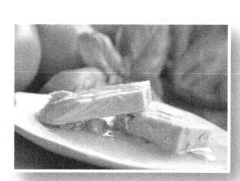

- ½ chunk light tuna, packed in water (preferable drained)
- 1 ½ cups lettuce greens
- ¾ cup other veggies
- Salad dressing (preferable low calories)

Directions:

1. Cut the vegetables. You can use ingredients like tomatoes, broccoli, onions, etc.
2. Place the salad vegetables on a plate.
3. Add the vegetables and tuna.
4. Pour the dressing on top.

Nutrition: Calories: 110 kcal; Protein: 24.2 g; Fat: 1.5 g; Carbs: 2.8 g.

91. Cucumber Yogurt

Serving: 3
Difficulty: 2
Preparation Time: 10 minutes
Cooking Time: 20 minutes
Optavia Counts: 1 lean/ 3 green/ 4 healthy fat/ 5 condiment
Ingredients:

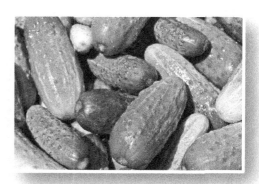

- 2 cups grated cucumbers
- ½ tsp. chili pepper
- ¼ cup parsley
- ¾ cup fresh dill
- 1 tbsp. lemon juice
- ½ tsp. salt
- ½ tsp. ground black pepper
- ¼ tsp. sage
- ½ tsp. oregano
- ⅓ cup Greek yogurt

Directions:

1. Make the cucumber dressing: puree the dill and parsley until you get a green paste.
2. Then mix the green puree with lemon juice, salt, ground black pepper, sage, oregano, Greek yogurt, and chili pepper.
3. Stir the mixture until well blended.
4. Roughly chop the cucumbers and mix them with the cucumber dressing. Mix well.
5. Place the cucumbers in the refrigerator for 20 minutes.

Nutrition: Calories: 114.8 kcal; Protein: 7.6 g; Fat: 1.6 g; Carbs: 23.2 g.

92. Lime Tarragon Dressing

Serving: 3
Difficulty: 1
Preparation Time: 10 minutes
Cooking Time: 0 minutes
Optavia Counts: 0 lean/ 0 green/ 1 healthy fat/ 8 condiment
Ingredients:

- 1 tbsp. oil
- 1 tsp. zero-calorie sugar substitute
- 1 tsp. dried tarragon
- 1 tbsp. lime juice
- Sea Salt and black pepper to taste
- 1 tbsp. balsamic vinegar
- ½ tbsp. dried chives
- 1 tsp. zero-calorie sugar substitute
- 1 garlic clove

Directions:

1. Mince the garlic. Squeeze juice from lime.
2. In a bowl, place all the ingredients and blend evenly.
3. Transfer the spiced composition in an air-tight jar.
4. Pour over salad or steamed vegetables.

Nutrition: Calories: 74 kcal; Protein: 0.5 g; Fat: 7 g; Carbs: 3.5 g.

93. Fantastic Salmon Salad

Serving: 3
Difficulty: 3
Preparation Time: 5 minutes
Cooking Time: 10 minutes
Optavia Counts: 1 lean/ 1 green/ 2 healthy fat/ 3 condiments
Ingredients:

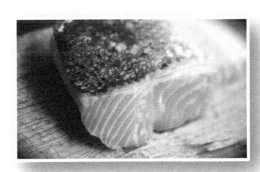

- 1 pound (500 g) salmon fillets
- 1 tbsp. soy sauce
- 8 zucchinis
- 1 tbsp. extra virgin olive oil
- 1 tbsp. sesame seeds
- Sea Salt
- Black Pepper

Directions:

1. Drizzle the salmon with soy sauce.
2. Heat a grill pan over medium flame.
3. Cook salmon on the grill on each side for 2-3 minutes.
4. Season the sliced zucchini with salt and pepper and place it on the grill as well.
5. Cook on each side until golden.
6. Place the zucchini, salmon, and the rest of the ingredients in a bowl.
7. Serve the salad fresh.

Nutrition: Calories: 224.18 kcal; Protein: 18.33 g; Fat: 19.10 g; Carbs: 0 g.

94. Juicy Fried Salmon

Serving: 4
Difficulty: 2
Preparation Time: 5 minutes
Cooking Time: 20 minutes
Optavia Counts: 1 lean/ 0 green/ 1 healthy fat/ 4 condiments
Ingredients:

- 4 (6-ounce) salmon fillets
- Sea Salt
- Black pepper
- 1 tsp. oregano
- 1 tsp. basil (preferable dried)
- 1 tbsp. Extra-virgin olive oil

Directions:

1. Season the fish with salt, pepper, oregano and basil.
2. Heat the oil in a pan and place the salmon, skin side down, in the hot oil.
3. Fry it for 2 minutes on each side until golden brown and fragrant.
4. Serve the salmon warm and fresh.

Nutrition: Calories: 327.1 kcal; Protein: 36.6 g; Fat: 25.8 g; Carbs: 0.31 g.

95. Salmon with Pineapple

Serving: 4
Difficulty: 3
Preparation Time: 5 minutes
Cooking Time: 30 minutes
Optavia Counts: 1 lean/ 1 green/ 1 healthy fat/ 8 condiments
Ingredients:

- 1 large salmon fillets
- Salt
- Black Pepper
- 1 tbsp. Cajun seasoning
- 17 fresh pineapple rings
- 1 cup cherry tomatoes
- 1 tbsp. cilantro
- 1 tbsp. parsley
- 1 tsp. mint (preferable dried)
- 1 tbsp. lemon juice
- 1 tbsp. olive oil
- 1 tsp. honey

Directions:

1. Season the fish with salt, pepper and Cajun seasoning. Peel and dice the pineapple.
2. Chop the cilantro and parsley. Quarter the cherry tomatoes.
3. Squeeze a lemon for the lemon juice.
4. Heat a grill pan over medium fire.
5. Cook fish on the grill for 3-4 minutes on each side.
6. For the salsa, combine the pineapple, tomatoes, cilantro, parsley, mint, lemon juice and honey in a bowl.
7. Season with salt and pepper.
8. Serve the grilled salmon with pineapple salsa.

Nutrition: Calories: 332 kcal; Protein: 34.10 g; Fat: 12.09 g; Carbs: 0 g.

96. Greek Fish

Serving: 4
Difficulty: 3
Preparation Time: 5 minutes
Cooking Time: 30 minutes
Optavia Counts: 1 lean/ 2 green/ 1 healthy fat/ 6 condiments
Ingredients:

- 4 salmon fillets
- 1 tbsp. oregano
- 1 tsp. basil (preferable dried)
- 1 zucchini
- 1 red onion
- 1 carrot
- 1 lemon
- 2 tbsp. olive oil
- Salt
- Black Pepper

Directions:

1. Chop the oregano. Slice the zucchini, the red onion, the carrot and the lemon.
2. Add all the ingredients to a deep-dish baking pan. Season with salt and pepper and cook it in the preheated oven at 350°F for 20 minutes. Serve the fish and vegetables warm.

Nutrition: Calories: 328.1 kcal; Protein: 38.8 g; Fat: 13.7 g; Carbs: 8 g.

97. Veggies and Fish Bake

Serving: 4
Difficulty: 3
Preparation Time: 5 minutes
Cooking Time: 30 minutes
Optavia Counts: 1 lean/ 3 green/ 1 healthy fat/ 4 condiments
Ingredients:

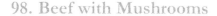

- Cod fillets
- Tomatoes
- Garlic cloves
- Shallot
- 1 celery stalk
- 1 tsp. fennel seeds
- 1 cup vegetable stock
- Salt
- Black Pepper

Directions:

1. Mince the garlic and slice the tomatoes, shallot and celery stalk. Layer the cod fillets and tomatoes in a deep-dish baking pan. Add the rest of the ingredients and add salt and pepper for the taste.
2. Cook in the preheated oven at 350F for 20 minutes. Serve the dish warm or chilled.

Nutrition: Calories: 299.1 kcal; Protein: 64.2 g; Fat: 3.28 g; Carbs: 2.01 g.

98. Beef with Mushrooms

Serving: 4
Difficulty: 5
Preparation Time: 5 minutes
Cooking Time: 8 hours
Optavia Counts: 1 lean/ 2 green/ 0 healthy fat/ 6 condiments
Ingredients:

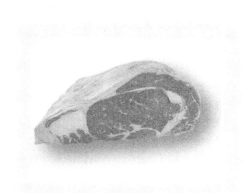

- 2 pounds beef
- ¼ cup balsamic vinegar
- 2 cups beef stock
- 1 tbsp. ginger
- Juice of ½ lemon
- 1 cup brown mushrooms.
- Sea salt
- Black pepper
- 1 tsp. ground cinnamon

Directions:

1. Cut the beef into strips. Peel and grate the ginger. Slice the mushrooms. Mix all the ingredients in your slow cooker, cover and cook on low for 8 hours. Divide everything among plates and serve.

Nutrition: Calories: 445.9 kcal; Protein: 70.8 g; Fat: 14.5 g; Carbs: 2.9 g.

CHAPTER 7.

SMOOTHIE RECIPES

99. Green Colada Smoothie

Servings: 1
Difficulty: 1
Preparation Time: 5 minutes
Cooking Time: 0 minutes
Optavia Counts: 0 lean/ 1 green/ 1 healthy fat/ 3 condiments
Ingredients:

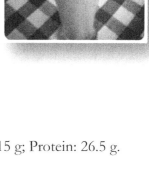

- 1 cup Greek yogurt
- 1 cup frozen pineapple
- 1 cup baby spinach
- ½ cup lite coconut milk
- ½ tsp. vanilla extract
- Coconut flakes for garnish

Directions:
1   Blend yogurt with pineapple, spinach, coconut milk, and vanilla in a blender until smooth.
2   Garnish with coconut flakes and serve.

Serving Suggestion: Enjoy this smoothie with breakfast muffins.
Variation Tip: Add some strawberries to the smoothie.
Nutrition: Calories: 325; Fat: 9 g; Sodium: 118 mg; Carbs: 35.4 g; Fiber: 2.9 g; Sugar: 15 g; Protein: 26.5 g.

100. Green Apple Smoothie

Servings: 1
Difficulty: 1
Preparation Time: 5 minutes
Cooking Time: 0 minutes
Optavia Counts: 0 lean/ 1 green/ 0 healthy fat/ 2 condiments
Ingredients:

- 2 ripe bananas
- 1 ripe pear, peeled, chopped
- 2 cups kale leaves, chopped
- ½ cup orange juice
- ½ cup cold water
- 12 ice cubes
- 1 tbsp. ground flaxseed

Directions:
1.   Blend bananas with pear, kale leaves, orange juice, cold water, ice cubes and flaxseed in a blender.
2.   Serve.

Serving Suggestion: Serve this smoothie with morning muffins.
Variation Tip: Add some strawberries to the smoothie.
Nutrition: Calories: 213; Fat: 2.5 g; Sodium: 15.6 mg; Carbs: 49.5 g; Fiber: 7.6 g; Sugar: 28 g; Protein: 3.5 g.

101. Refreshing Lime Smoothie

Servings: 1
Difficulty: 1
Preparation Time: 10 minutes
Cooking Time: 0 minutes
Optavia Counts: 0 lean/ 1 green/ 2 healthy fat/ 5 condiments
Ingredients:

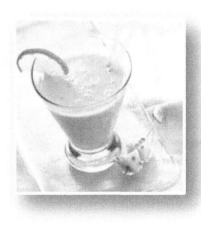

- 1 cup ice cubes
- 20 drops liquid stevia
- 1 tbsp. fresh lime, peeled and halved
- 1 tbsp. lime zest, grated
- ½ cucumber, chopped
- 1 avocado, pitted and peeled
- 1 cup fresh spinach
- 1 tbsp. creamed coconut
- ¾ cup coconut water

Directions:

1. Add all ingredients to the blender and blend until smooth and creamy.
2. Serve immediately and enjoy.

Nutrition: Calories: 312; Fat: 3 g; Carbs: 28 3 g; Protein: 4 g.

102. Broccoli Green Smoothie

Servings: 1
Difficulty: 1
Preparation Time: 10 minutes
Cooking Time: 0 minutes
Optavia Counts: 0 lean/ 3 green/ 0 healthy fat/ 0 condiments
Ingredients:

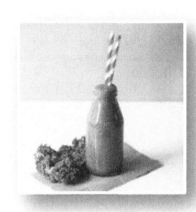

- celery, peeled and chopped
- 1 lemon, peeled
- 1 apple, diced
- 1 banana
- 1 cup spinach
- ½ cup broccoli

Directions:

1. Add all ingredients to the blender and blend until smooth and creamy.
2. Serve immediately and enjoy.

Nutrition: Calories: 121; Fat: 1 g; Carbs: 18 g; Protein: 1 g.

103. Apple Spinach Cucumber Smoothie

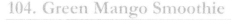

Servings: 1
Difficulty: 1
Preparation Time: 10 minutes
Cooking Time: 0 minutes
Optavia Counts: 0 lean/ 1 green/ 0 healthy fat/ 0 condiments
Ingredients:

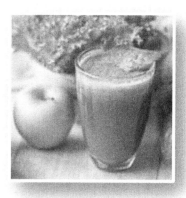

- ¾ cup water
- ½ green apple, diced
- ¾ cup spinach
- ½ cucumber

Directions:

1. Add all ingredients to the blender and blend until smooth and creamy.
2. Serve immediately and enjoy.

Nutrition: Calories: 90; Fat: 1 g; Carbs: 21 g; Protein: 1 g.

104. Green Mango Smoothie

Servings: 1
Difficulty: 1
Preparation Time: 5 minutes
Cooking Time: 0 minutes
Optavia Counts: 0 lean/ 1 green/ 0 healthy fat/ 0 condiments
Ingredients:

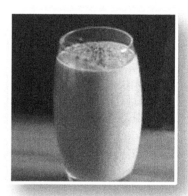

- 2 cups spinach
- 1-2 cups coconut water
- 2 mangos, ripe, peeled & diced

Directions:

1. Blend everything together until smooth.

Nutrition: Calories: 120; Fat: 1 g; Carbs: 5 g; Protein: 8 g.

105. Sweet Green Smoothie

Servings: 1
Difficulty: 1
Preparation Time: 10 minutes
Cooking Time: 0 minutes
Optavia Counts: 0 lean/ 0 green/ 0 healthy fat/ 3 condiments
Ingredients:

- 1 tbsp. flax seeds
- ½ cup wheatgrass
- 1 1/2 cups mango pieces
- 1 cup pomegranate juice

Directions:

1. Add all ingredients to the blender and blend until smooth and creamy.
2. Serve immediately and enjoy.

Nutrition: Calories: 177; Fat: 1 g, Carbs: 21 g; Protein: 5 g.

106. Super Healthy Green Smoothie

Servings: 2
Difficulty: 1
Preparation Time: 10 minutes
Cooking Time: 0 minutes
Optavia Counts: 0 lean/ 4 green/ 1 healthy fat/ 2 condiments
Ingredients:

- 1 tsp. spirulina powder
- 1 cup coconut water
- 2 cups mixed greens
- 1 tbsp. ginger
- 1 tbsp. lemon juice
- 4 celery stalks
- 1 cup cucumber, chopped
- 1 green pear, core removed
- 1 banana

Directions:

1. Add all ingredients to the blender and blend until smooth and creamy.
2. Serve immediately and enjoy.

Nutrition: Calories: 161; Fat: 1 g; Carbs: 19 g; Protein: 7 g.

107. Spinach Smoothie

Servings: 2
Difficulty: 1
Preparation Time: 5 minutes
Cooking Time: 0 minutes
Optavia Counts: 0 lean/ 1 green/ 1 healthy fat/ 2 condiments
Ingredients:

- 1 cup fresh spinach
- 1 banana
- ½ green apple
- 6 oz fresh hulled strawberries
- ½ cup frozen mango chunks
- ⅓ cup whole milk
- 1 scoop vanilla protein powder
- 1 tsp. honey

Directions:

1. Blend spinach with banana with the green apple with strawberries, mango, milk, protein powder and honey in a blender.
2. Serve.

Serving Suggestion: Enjoy this smoothie with breakfast muffins.
Variation Tip: Add some blueberries to the smoothie.
Nutrition: Calories: 312; Fat: 25 g; Sodium: 132 mg; Carbs: 44 g; Fiber: 3.9 g; Sugar: 3 g; Protein: 18.9 g.

108. Spinach Peach Banana Smoothie

Servings: 2
Difficulty: 1
Preparation Time: 10 minutes
Cooking Time: 0 minutes
Optavia Counts: 0 lean/ 1 green/ 0 healthy fat/ 2 condiments
Ingredients:

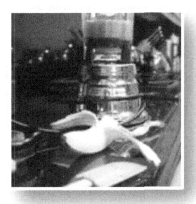

- 1 cup baby spinach
- 8 ounces unsweetened coconut water
- 1 tbsp. agave syrup
- 1 medium ripe bananas
- 1 cup ripe peaches, pitted and chopped

Directions:

1. Add all ingredients to the blender and blend until smooth and creamy.
2. Serve immediately and enjoy.

Nutrition: Calories: 163; Fat: 1 g; Carbs: 4 g; Protein: 6 g.

109. Spinach Coconut Smoothie

Servings: 2
Difficulty: 1
Preparation Time: 10 minutes
Cooking Time: 0 minutes
Optavia Counts: 0 lean/ 1 green/ 1 healthy fat/ 2 condiments
Ingredients:

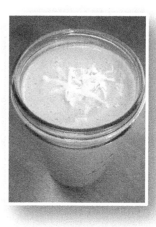

- 1 tbsp. unsweetened coconut flakes
- 2 cups fresh pineapple
- ½ cup coconut water
- 1 and ½ cups coconut milk
- 2 cups fresh spinach

Directions:

1. Add all ingredients to the blender and blend until smooth and creamy.
2. Serve immediately and enjoy.

Nutrition: Calories: 290; Fat: 1 g; Carbs: 22g; Protein: 8 g.

110. Salty Green Smoothie

Servings: 2
Difficulty: 1
Preparation Time: 10 minutes
Cooking Time: 0 minutes
Optavia Counts: 0 lean/ 3 green/ 1 healthy fat/ 3 condiments
Ingredients:

- 1 cup ice cubes
- ¼ tbsp. liquid aminos
- 1 and ½ tbsp. sea salt
- 2 limes, peeled and quartered
- 1 avocado, pitted and peeled
- 1 cup kale leaves
- 1 cucumber, chopped
- 2 cups tomato, chopped
- ¼ cup water

Directions:

1. Add all ingredients to the blender and blend until smooth and creamy.
2. Serve immediately and enjoy.

Nutrition: Calories: 108; Fat: 1 g; Carbs: 1 g; Protein: 4 g.

111. Watermelon Strawberry Smoothie

Servings: 2
Difficulty: 1
Preparation Time: 10 minutes
Cooking Time: 0 minutes
Optavia Counts: 0 lean/ 0 green/ 1 healthy fat/ 0 condiments
Ingredients:

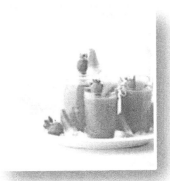

- 1 cup coconut milk yogurt
- ½ cup strawberries
- 4 cups fresh watermelon
- 1 banana

Directions:

1. Toss all your ingredients into your blender, then process until smooth.
2. Serve and enjoy.

Nutrition: Calories: 160; Fat: 1 g; Carbs: 3 g; Protein: 4 g.

112. Avocado Mango Smoothie

Servings: 2
Difficulty: 1
Preparation Time: 10 minutes
Cooking Time: 0 minutes
Optavia Counts: 0 lean/ 1 green/ 1 healthy fat/ 1 condiments
Ingredients:

- 1 cup ice cubes
- ½ cup mango
- ½ avocado
- 1 tbsp. ginger
- kale leaves
- 1 cup coconut water

Directions:

1. Toss all your ingredients into your blender, then process until smooth.
2. Serve and enjoy.

Nutrition: Calories: 290; Fat: 3 g; Carbs: 18 g; Protein: 11 g.

113. Chia Seed Smoothie

Servings: 3
Difficulty: 1
Preparation Time: 5 minutes
Cooking Time: 0 minutes
Optavia Counts: 0 lean/ 1 green/ 1 healthy fat/ 6 condiments
Ingredients:

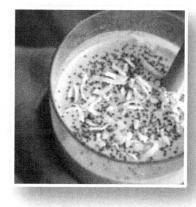

- ¼ teaspoon cinnamon
- 1 tablespoon ginger, fresh & grated
- ¼ teaspoon ground cardamom
- 1 tablespoon chia seeds
- 2 medjool dates, pitted
- 1 cup alfalfa sprouts
- 1 cup water
- 1 banana
- ½ cup coconut milk, unsweetened

Directions:

1. Blend everything together until smooth.

Nutrition: Calories: 412; Protein: 18.9 g; Carbs: 43.8 g; Fat: 24.8 g.

114. Matcha Avocado Smoothie

Servings: 3
Difficulty: 1
Preparation Time: 5 minutes
Cooking Time: 0 minutes
Optavia Counts: 0 lean/ 2 green/ 3 healthy fat/ 4 condiments
Ingredients:

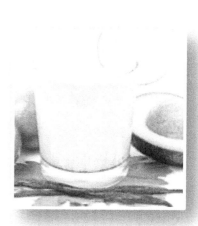

- ½ avocado, peeled and cubed
- ⅓ cucumber
- 2 cups spinach
- 1 cup coconut milk
- 1 cup almond milk
- 1 tsp. matcha powder
- ½ lime juice
- ½ scoop vanilla protein powder
- ½ tsp. chia seeds

Directions:

1. Blend avocado flesh with cucumber and the rest of the ingredients in a blender until smooth.
2. Serve.

Serving Suggestion: Enjoy this smoothie with breakfast muffins.
Variation Tip: Add some strawberries to the smoothie.
Nutrition: Calories: 297; Fat: 15 g; Sodium: 202 mg; Carbs: 58.5 g; Fiber: 4 g; Sugar: 1 g; Protein: 7.3 g.

115. Healthy Green Smoothie

Servings: 3
Difficulty: 1
Preparation Time: 10 minutes
Cooking Time: 0 minutes
Optavia Counts: 0 lean/ 1 green/ 1 healthy fat/ 0 condiments
Ingredients:

- 1 cup water
- 1 fresh lemon, peeled
- 1 avocado
- 1 cucumber, peeled
- 1 cup spinach
- 1 cup ice cubes

Directions:

1. Add all ingredients to the blender and blend until smooth and creamy.
2. Serve immediately and enjoy.

Nutrition: Calories: 160; Fat: 13 g; Carbs: 12 g; Protein: 2 g.

116. Mango Smoothie

Servings: 3
Difficulty: 1
Preparation Time: 5 minutes
Cooking Time: 0 minutes
Servings: 3
Optavia Counts: 0 lean/ 1 green/ 0 healthy fat/ 0 condiments
Ingredients:

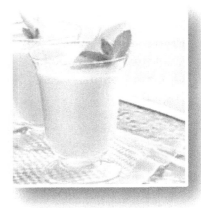

- 1 carrot, peeled & chopped
- 1 cup strawberries
- 1 cup water
- 1 cup peaches, chopped
- 1 banana, frozen & sliced
- 1 cup mango, chopped

Directions:

1. Blend everything together until smooth.

Nutrition: Calories: 221; Fat: 1 g; Carbs: 5 g; Protein: 4 g.

117. Watermelon Kale Smoothie

Servings: 3
Difficulty: 1
Preparation Time: 10 minutes
Cooking Time: 0 minutes
Optavia Counts: 0 lean/ 2 green/ 0 healthy fat/ 0 condiments
Ingredients:

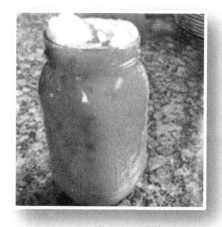

- ½ cup water
- 1 orange, peeled
- 2 cups kale, chopped
- 1 banana, peeled
- 2 cups watermelon, chopped
- 1 celery, chopped

Directions:

1. Add all ingredients to the blender and blend until smooth and creamy.
2. Serve immediately and enjoy.

Nutrition: Calories: 122; Fat: 1 g; Carbs: 5 g; Protein: 1 g.

118. Mix Berry Watermelon Smoothie

Servings: 3
Difficulty: 1
Preparation Time: 10 minutes
Cooking Time: 0 minutes
Optavia Counts: 0 lean/ 1 green/ 0 healthy fat/ 1 condiments
Ingredients:

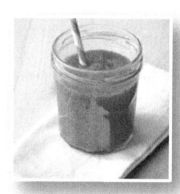

- 1 cup alkaline water
- ¼ cup fresh lemon juices
- ¼ cup fresh mint leaves
- 1 ½ cups mixed berries
- 2 cups watermelon

Directions:

1. Toss all your ingredients into your blender, then process until smooth. Serve immediately and enjoy.

Nutrition: Calories: 188; Fat: 1 g; Carbs: 2 g; Protein: 1 g.

119. Plum and Avocado Smoothie

Servings: 4
Difficulty: 4
Preparation Time: 2 hours
Cooking Time: 0 minutes
Optavia Counts: 0 lean/ 0 green/ 2 healthy fat/ 4 condiments
Ingredients:

- 1 cup avocado, peeled, pitted, and chopped
- 1 cup plums, chopped
- 1 cup almond milk
- 3 drops stevia
- 1 tsp. vanilla extract
- 1 tsp. lemon juice

Directions:

1. In a blender, combine the avocado with the plums and the rest of the ingredients, blend, divide into glasses and keep in the fridge for 2 hours before serving.

Nutrition: Calories: 148; Fat: 3,3 g; Carbs: 39,4 g; Fiber: 4,3 g; Protein: 1,5 g.

120. Creamy Raspberry Pomegranate Smoothie

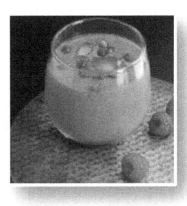

Servings: 4
Difficulty: 1
Preparation Time: 5 minutes
Cooking Time: 5 minutes
Optavia Counts: 0 lean/ 1 green/ 1 healthy fat/ 2 condiments
Ingredients:

- 1 ½ cups pomegranate juice
- ½ cup unsweetened coconut milk
- 1 scoop vanilla protein powder (plant-based if you need it to be dairy-free)
- ¼ cup fresh baby spinach
- 1 cup frozen raspberries
- 1 frozen banana
- 1 to 2 tbsp. freshly compressed lemon juice

Directions:

1. In a blender, combine the pomegranate juice and coconut milk. Add the protein powder and spinach. Give these a whirl to break down the spinach.
2. Add the raspberries, banana, and lemon juice, then top it off with ice. Blend until smooth and frothy.

Nutrition: Calories: 303; Total fat: 3 g; Cholesterol: 0 mg; Fiber: 2 g; Protein: 15 g; Sodium: 165 mg.

121. Lean and Green Smoothie 1

Servings: 4
Difficulty: 1
Preparation Time: 5 minutes
Cooking Time: 0 minutes
Optavia Counts: 0 lean/ 1 green/ 0 healthy fat/ 0 condiments
Ingredients:

- ½ cups of kale leaves
- ¾ cup of chilled apple juice
- 1 cup of cubed pineapple
- ½ cup of frozen green grapes
- ½ cup of chopped apple

Directions:

1. Place the pineapple, apple juice, apple, frozen seedless grapes, and kale leaves in a blender.
2. Cover and blend until it's smooth.
3. Smoothie is ready and can be garnished with halved grapes if you wish.

Nutrition: Calories: 81; Protein: 2 g; Carbs: 19 g; Fats: 1 g.

122. Pumpkin Smoothie

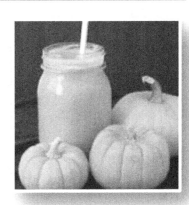

Servings: 4
Difficulty: 1
Preparation Time: 5 minutes
Cooking Time: 0 minutes
Optavia Counts: 0 lean/ 0 green/ 4 healthy fat/ 2 condiments
Ingredients:

- 1 tbsp. whipped topping
- 1 tbsp. pumpkin puree
- 1 tbsp. MCT oil
- ½ cup almond milk, unsweetened
- ½ cup coconut milk, unsweetened
- ½ tsp. pumpkin pie spice
- 1 ½ cups crushed ice

Directions:

1. Place all the ingredients in the order into a food processor or blender, and then pulse for 2 to 3 minutes until smooth.
2. Distribute smoothie between two glasses and then serve.

Nutrition: Calories 285 Fats 27 g; Protein 2.1 g; Net Carb 6.2 g; Fiber 1.6 g

CHAPTER 8.

FISH AND SEAFOOD RECIPES

123. Dill Relish on White Sea Bass

Servings: 1
Difficulty: 1
Preparation Time: 10 minutes
Cooking Time: 12 minutes
Optavia Counts: 1 lean/ 1 green/ 0 healthy fat/ 4 condiments
Ingredients:
- 1 tsp. lemon juice - 1 tsp. Dijon mustard
- 1 ½ tsp. chopped fresh dill
- 1 tsp. pickled baby capers, drained
- 1 ½ tbsp. chopped white onion
- 1 lemon, quartered
- 4 pieces (4-oz.) white sea bass fillets

Directions:
1. Preheat oven to 375°F.
2. Mix lemon juice, mustard, dill, capers, and onions in a small bowl. Prepare 4 aluminum foil squares and place 1 fillet per foil.
3. Squeeze a lemon wedge per fish. Evenly divide into 4 the dill spread and drizzle over the fillet.
4. Close the foil over the fish securely and pop it in the oven. Bake for 12 minutes or until fish is cooked through.
5. Remove from foil and transfer to a serving platter.

Nutrition: Calories: 115; Protein: 7 g; Fat: 1 g; Carbohydrate: 12 g.

124. Summer Shrimp Primavera

Servings: 1
Difficulty: 1
Preparation Time: 10 minutes
Cooking Time: 10 minutes
Optavia Counts: 1 lean/ 3 green/ 2 healthy fat/ 5 condiments
Ingredients:

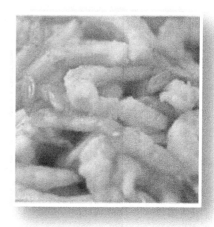

- 4 oz. uncooked angel hair pasta
- 8 shrimp jumbos, peeled and deveined
- ¼ tsp. salt
- ⅛ tsp. crushed red pepper flakes
- 6 fresh asparagus spears, cut into 2-inch pieces
- ¼ cup olive oil - 2 garlic cloves, minced
- ½ cup fresh sliced mushrooms
- ½ cup chicken broth
- 1 tiny, peeled, seeded, and diced plum tomato
- 1 tbsp. fresh basil, oregano, thyme, and parsley each
- ¼ cup grated Parmesan cheese

Directions:
1. In a big saucepan, cook pasta according to package directions for al-dente pasta; drain.
2. Preheat broiler. Spray a broiler-proof baking dish with nonstick spray. Sprinkle shrimp with salt and pepper. Arrange on a metal baking pan coated with nonstick spray. Broil for 2 minutes, 4 inches from the sun. Turn shrimp and broil for 2 minutes longer or until done.
3. Cook the pasta until tender in boiling water (1 to 2 minutes). Run under cold water, drain well, and keep warm.
4. In a big/large non-stick skillet, heat the olive oil over medium-high fire. Add the garlic, asparagus, mushrooms, tomato, and chicken broth; heat through. Stir in the pasta and shrimp; cook until it is completely ready. Season with salt and pepper flakes. Stir herbs into shrimp mixture. Sprinkle with cheese. Serve immediately.

Nutrition: Calories: 291; Protein: 20.7 g; Fat: 17.84 g; Carbs: 12.43 g; Calcium: 100 mg; Magnesium: 39 mg; Phosphorus: 229 mg.

125. Grilled Salmon with Cucumber Dill Sauce

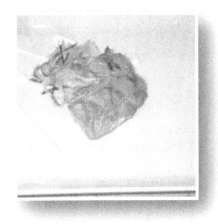

Servings: 1
Difficulty: 2
Preparation Time: 40 minutes
Cooking Time: 25 minutes
Optavia Counts: 1 lean/ 1 green/ 2 healthy fat/ 5 condiments
Ingredients:

- 4 (6-oz) salmon fillets
- Salt and pepper to taste
- 1 tsp. smoked paprika
- 1 tsp. dried sage
- 1 cucumbers, sliced
- 1 tbsp. chopped dill
- ½ cup Greek yogurt
- 1 tbsp. lemon juice
- 1 tbsp. olive oil

Directions:

1. Season the salmon with salt, pepper, paprika, and sage.
2. Heat a grill pan over medium flame and place the salmon on the grill.
3. Cook on each side for 4 minutes.
4. For the sauce, mix the cucumbers, dill, yogurt, lemon juice, and oil in a bowl. Add salt and pepper and mix well.
5. Serve the salmon with cucumber sauce.

Nutrition: Calories: 224; Fat: 10 g; Protein: 26.3 g; Carbohydrate: 8.9 g.

126. Shrimp and Endives

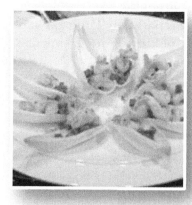

Servings: 2
Difficulty: 1
Preparation Time: 5 minutes
Cooking Time: 12 minutes
Optavia Counts: 1 lean/ 2 green/ 1 healthy fat/ 3 condiments
Ingredients:

- 1 pound shrimp, peeled and deveined
- 1 tbsp. avocado oil
- 1 spring onions, chopped
- 4-6 endives, shredded
- 1 tbsp. balsamic vinegar
- 1 tbsp. chives, minced
- A pinch of sea salt and black pepper

Directions:

1. Over medium-high flame, heat a pan with the oil, add the spring onions, endives, and chives. Stir and cook for 4 minutes.
2. Add the shrimp and remaining ingredients. Toss and cook for 8 more minutes over medium heat, divide into bowls and serve.

Nutrition: Calories: 378; Fat: 2 g; Carbohydrate: 6 g; Protein: 6 g; Sodium: 290 mg.

127. Basil 'n Lime-Chili Clams

Servings: 2
Difficulty: 1
Preparation Time: 5 minutes
Cooking Time: 15 minutes
Optavia Counts: 1 lean/ 2 green/ 1 healthy fat/ 3 condiments
Ingredients:

- ½ cup basil leaves
- ½ cup tomatoes, chopped
- 1 tbsp. fresh lime juice
- 25 littleneck clams
- 1 garlic cloves, minced
- 1 tbsp. unsalted butter
- Salt and pepper to taste

Directions:

1. Preheat the Air Fryer to 390°F.
2. Put the grill pan accessory in the Air Fryer.
3. On a large foil, place all ingredients. Fold over the foil and close by crimping the edges.
4. Put on the grill pan and cook for 15 minutes.
5. Serve with bread.

Nutrition: Calories: 163; Carbs: 4.1 g; Protein: 1.7 g; Fat: 15.5 g.

128. Baked Fish Fillets

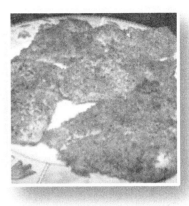

Servings: 2
Difficulty: 1
Preparation Time: 5 minutes
Cooking Time: 20 minutes
Optavia Counts: 1 lean/ 0 green/ 1 healthy fat/ 4 condiments
Ingredients:

- 1 tbsp. butter, melted
- A pinch of ground paprika
- 1 fish fillets (5 oz.)
- Pepper to taste
- 1 tbsp. lemon juice
- ½ tsp. salt

Directions:

1. Ensure that your oven is preheated to 350°F. By greasing it with some fat, prepare a pan for baking.
2. Sprinkle the fillets with salt and pepper and put them in the pan.
3. In a bowl, add the butter, paprika, and lemon juice and stir.
4. Brush over the fillets with this mixture.
5. In the oven, put the baking pan and cook the fillets.

Nutrition: Calories: 245; Fat: 12 g; Carbohydrate: 4 g; Protein: 32 g; Sodium: 455 mg.

129. Grilled Split Lobster

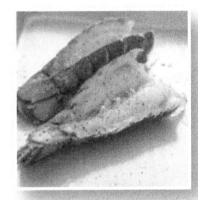

Servings: 2
Difficulty: 1
Preparation Time: 10 minutes
Cooking Time: 15 minutes
Optavia Counts: 1 lean/ 0 green/ 2 healthy fat/ 4 condiments
Ingredients:

- 1 tbsp. olive oil or melted butter
- 1 tbsp. Kosher salt to taste
- 4 live lobsters (1½ pounds each)
- Freshly ground pepper to taste
- Melted butter to serve
- Hot sauce like Frank's hot sauce, to serve
- Lemon wedges to serve

Directions:

1. For 15 minutes, put the live lobsters in the freezer.
2. Place them on your cutting board with the belly down. Hold the tail. Split the lobsters in half lengthwise. Start from the point where the tail joins the body and goes up to the head. Flip sides and cut it lengthwise via the tail.
3. Rub melted butter on the cut part immediately after cutting it. Sprinkle salt and pepper over it.
4. Set up your grill and preheat it to high heat for 5–10 minutes. Clean the grill grate and lower the heat to low heat.
5. Place the lobsters on the grill and press the claws on the grill until cooked—grill for 6–8 minutes.
6. Flip sides and cook until it is cooked through and lightly charred.
7. Transfer to a plate. Drizzle melted butter on top and serve.

Nutrition: Calories: 433; Fat: 4 g; Carbohydrate: 26 g; Protein: 6 g; Sodium: 455 mg.

130. Fish Bone Broth

Servings: 2
Difficulty: 5
Preparation Time: 10 minutes
Cooking Time: 4 hours
Optavia Counts: 1 lean/ 0 green/ 0 healthy fat/ 3 condiments
Ingredients:

- 2 1/2 to 3 pounds fish head or carcass
- Salt to taste
- 7–8 quarts water + extra to blanch
- 2 inches ginger, sliced
- 1 tbsp. lemon juice

Directions:

1. To blanch the fish: Add water and fish heads into a large pot. Place the pot over high heat.
2. Turn the heat off when it boils and discard the water.
3. Place the fish back in the pot. Pour 7–8 quarts of water.
4. Place the pot over high heat. Add ginger, salt, and lemon juice.
5. Reduce the heat as the mixture boils, and cover it with a lid.
6. Remove from heat. When it cools down, strain into a large jar with a wire mesh strainer.
7. Refrigerate for 5–6 days. Unused broth can be frozen.

Nutrition: Calories: 254; Fat: 4 g; Carbohydrate: 26 g; Protein: 6 g; Sodium: 455 mg.

131. Salmon Cakes

Servings: 2
Difficulty: 1
Preparation Time: 10 minutes
Cooking Time: 10 minutes
Optavia Counts: 2 lean/ 0 green/ 1 healthy fat/ 5 condiments
Ingredients:

- 2 cans salmon (14.75 oz. each), drained
- 1 tbsp. collagen
- 2 cups shredded mozzarella cheese
- 1 tsp. onion powder
- 1 large pastured eggs
- 1 tsp. dried dill
- 1 tsp.pink sea salt or to taste
- 1 tbsp. bacon grease

Directions:

1. Add salmon, collagen, mozzarella, onion powder, eggs, dill, and salt into a bowl and mix well.
2. Make 8 patties from the mixture. Place a large skillet with bacon grease over a medium-low flame.
3. Place the salmon cakes in the skillet once the fat is well heated and cook until it becomes golden brown on all sides. Take off the pan from heat and let the patties remain in the cooked fat for 5 minutes. Serve.

Nutrition: Calories: 204; Fat: 10 g; Carbohydrate: 5 g; Protein: 29 g; Sodium: 643 mg.

132. Lemon Aioli and Swordfish Panini

Servings: 3
Difficulty: 1
Preparation Time: 25 minutes
Cooking Time: 15 minutes
Optavia Counts: 1 lean/ 1 green/ 1 healthy fat/ 3 condiments
Ingredients:
Swordfish Panini:

- 2 oz. fresh arugula greens
- 1 loaf focaccia bread
- 2 garlic cloves minced
- 1 tbsp. herbs de Provence
- Pepper and salt
- 4 pieces (6-oz.) swordfish fillet
- 1 ½ tbsp. olive oil

Lemon Aioli:

- ¼ tsp. freshly ground black pepper
- ¼ tsp. salt
- 2 clove garlic, minced
- 1 tbsp. fresh lemon juice
- 1 lemon, zested
- ⅔ cup mayonnaise

Directions:

1. In a small bowl, mix well all lemon aioli ingredients and put them aside.
2. Over medium-high fire, heat olive oil in a skillet. Season the swordfish with pepper, salt, minced garlic, and herbs de Provence. Then pan-fry fish until golden brown on both sides, around 5 minutes per side.
3. Slice bread into four slices. Smear on the lemon aioli mixture on two bread slices, layer with arugula leaves and fried fish; then cover with the remaining bread slices before grilling in a Panini press.
4. Grill until bread is crisped and ridged.

Nutrition: Calories: 433; Carbohydrate: 15 g; Protein: 36.2 g; Fat: 25 g.

133. Salmon with Mustard

Servings: 3
Difficulty: 1
Preparation Time: 10 minutes
Cooking Time: 8 minutes
Optavia Counts: 1 lean/ 0 green/ 0 healthy fat/ 7 condiments
Ingredients:

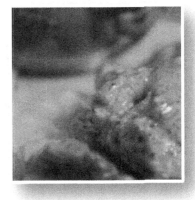

- ¼ tsp. ground red pepper or chili powder
- ¼ tsp. ground turmeric
- ¼ tsp. salt
- 1 tsp. honey
- ⅛ tsp. garlic powder or a minced garlic clove
- 1 tsp. wholegrain mustard
- 1 ½ lb salmon fillets
- Cooking spray

Directions:

1. In a small bowl, mix well salt, garlic powder, red pepper, turmeric, honey, and mustard.
2. Preheat the oven to broil and grease a baking dish with cooking spray.
3. Place salmon on a baking dish with skin side down and spread the mustard mixture evenly on top of salmon. Pop in the oven and broil until flaky, around 8 minutes.

Nutrition: Calories: 324; Fat: 18.9 g; Protein: 34 g; Carbs: 2.9 g.

134. Dijon Mustard and Lime Marinated Shrimp

Servings: 3
Difficulty: 1
Preparation Time: 10 minutes
Cooking Time: 10 minutes
Optavia Counts: 1 lean/ 0 green/ 0 healthy fat/ 8 condiments
Ingredients:

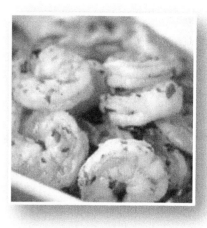

- ½ cup fresh lime juice and lime zest as garnish
- ½ cup rice vinegar
- ½ tsp. hot sauce
- 6 bay leaves
- 1 cup water
- 1 pound uncooked shrimp, peeled and deveined
- 1 medium red onion, chopped
- 1 tbsp. capers
- 1 tbsp. Dijon mustard
- 3 whole cloves

Directions:

1. Mix hot sauce, mustard, capers, lime juice, and onion in a shallow baking dish and set aside.
2. Put the bay leaf, cloves, vinegar, and water to a boil in a large saucepan.
3. Once boiling, add shrimps and cook for a minute while stirring continuously.
4. Drain shrimps and pour them into the onion mixture. For an hour, refrigerate and cover the shrimps.
5. Then serve shrimps cold and garnished with lime zest.

Nutrition: Calories: 232.2; Protein: 17.8 g; Fat: 3 g; Carbs: 15 g.

135. Breaded and Spiced Halibut

Servings: 3
Difficulty: 1
Preparation Time: 15 minutes
Cooking Time: 20 minutes
Optavia Counts: 1 lean/ 3 green/ 1 healthy fat/ 4 condiments
Ingredients:

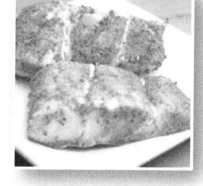

- ¼ tsp. ground black pepper
- 1 tsp. sea salt
- 1 tsp. finely grated lemon zest
- 1 tbsp. extra-virgin olive oil
- ¼ cup chopped fresh chives
- ¼ cup chopped fresh dill
- ⅓ cup chopped fresh parsley
- ¾ cup panko breadcrumbs
- 2 pieces (8-oz.) halibut fillets

Directions:

1. Line a baking sheet with foil, grease with cooking spray, and preheat the oven to 400°F.
2. In a small bowl, mix black pepper, sea salt, lemon zest, olive oil, chives, dill, parsley, and breadcrumbs. If needed, add more salt to taste. Set aside. Meanwhile, wash halibut fillets on cold tap water. Dry with paper towels and place on a prepared baking sheet. Generously spoon crumb mixture onto halibut fillets. Ensure that fillets are covered with crumb mixture. Press down on crumb mixture onto each fillet. Pop into the oven and bake for 10–15 minutes or until fish is flaky and the crumb topping is already lightly browned.

Nutrition: Calories: 336; Protein: 25 g; Fat: 25 g; Carbohydrate: 4 g.

136. Cilantro Shrimp

Servings: 3
Difficulty: 1
Preparation Time: 10 minutes
Cooking Time: 15 minutes
Optavia Counts: 1 lean/ 1 green/ 2 healthy fat/ 2 condiments
Ingredients:

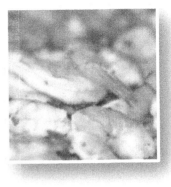

- 1-pound shrimps
- 3 garlic cloves, diced
- ¼ cup fresh cilantro, chopped
- 1 tbsp. butter
- ¼ cup milk - ½ tsp. salt

Directions:

1. Put butter in the skillet and bring it to a boil. Then add diced garlic and roast it for 3 minutes. Add milk and salt. Bring the liquid to a boil (it will take about 2 minutes). After this, add shrimps and mix up well. Cook the shrimps for 3 minutes over medium heat. Then add fresh cilantro. Close the lid and cook seafood for 5 minutes. Serve the cooked garlic shrimps with cilantro-garlic sauce.

Nutrition: Calories: 197; Fat: 8 g; Fiber: 0.1 g; Carbohydrate: 3.3 g; Protein: 26.6 g.

137. Garlicky Clams

Servings: 3
Difficulty: 1
Preparation Time: 5 minutes
Cooking Time: 10 minutes
Optavia Counts: 1 lean/ 0 green/ 1 healthy fat/ 4 condiments
Ingredients:

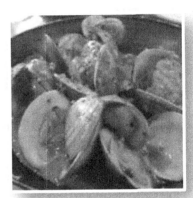

- 4 pounds clams, clean
- 5 garlic cloves
- ½ cup olive oil
- ½ cup fresh lemon juice
- 1 cup white wine
- Pepper Salt to taste

Directions:

1. Add oil into the inner pot of the instant pot and set the pot on sauté mode.
2. Add garlic and sauté for 1 minute.
3. Add clams and cook for 2 minutes.
4. Add remaining ingredients and stir well.
5. Seal pot with a lid and cook on High for 2 minutes.
6. Once done, allow to release pressure naturally. Remove lid. Serve and enjoy.

Nutrition: Calorie 332; Fat: 13.5 g; Carbohydrate: 40.5 g; Sugar: 12.5 g; Protein: 2.5 g; Cholesterol: 0 mg.

138. Lemon Swordfish

Servings: 3
Difficulty: 1
Preparation Time: 6 minutes
Cooking Time: 10 minutes
Optavia Counts: 1 lean/ 0 green/ 0 healthy fat/ 4 condiments
Ingredients:

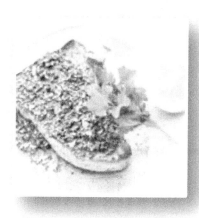

- 12 oz. swordfish steaks (6 oz. every fish steak)
- 1 tsp. ground cumin
- 1 tbsp. lemon juice
- ¼ tsp. salt
- 1 tsp. olive oil

Directions:

1. Sprinkle the fish steaks with ground cumin and salt from each side.
2. Then drizzle the lemon juice over the steaks and massage them gently with your fingertips.
3. Preheat the grill to 395°F.
4. Brush every fish steak with olive oil and place it in the drill.
5. Cook the swordfish for 3 minutes from each side.

Nutrition: Calories: 289; Fat: 1.5 g; Fiber: 0.1 g; Carbohydrate: 0.6 g; Protein: 43.4 g.

139. Baked Scallops with Garlic Aioli

Servings: 4
Difficulty: 1
Preparation Time: 5 minutes
Cooking Time: 10 minutes
Optavia Counts: 1 lean/ 1 green/ 2 healthy fat/ 5 condiments
Ingredients:

- 2 shallots, chopped
- 5 garlic cloves, minced
- 1 tbsp. butter, melted
- 16 sea scallops, rinsed and drained
- Salt and pepper to taste
- 3 pinches ground nutmeg
- 1 tbsp. olive oil - 1 cup breadcrumbs
- ¼ cup chopped parsley

Directions:

1. Grease baking pan of Air Fryer with cooking spray. Mix in shallots, garlic, melted butter, and scallops. Season with pepper, salt, and nutmeg. In a small bowl, whisk well olive oil and breadcrumbs. Sprinkle over scallops. For 10 minutes, cook on 390°F until tops are lightly browned.
2. Serve and enjoy with a sprinkle of parsley.

Nutrition: Calories: 452; Carbohydrate: 29.8 g; Protein: 15.2 g; Fat: 30.2 g.

140. Tilapia Tacos

Servings: 4
Difficulty: 1
Preparation Time: 10 minutes
Cooking Time: 16 minutes
Optavia Counts: 1 lean/ 1 green/ 3 healthy fat/ 6 condiments
Ingredients:

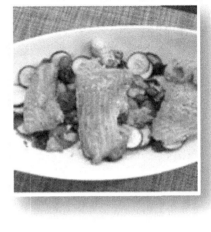

- ⅓ cup sour cream
- ¾ cup Pace Chunky Salsa
- ⅛ tsp. chipotle chili powder
- 4 tilapia fillets
- ¼ tsp. salt
- ¼ tsp. black pepper
- ½ tsp. cumin
- 1 tbsp. canola oil
- 1 tsp. lime juice
- 8 warmed flour tortilla (6-inch)
- 1 cup shredded red cabbage

Directions:

1. In a shallow bowl, whisk the sour cream, ¼ cup salsa, and the chipotle chili powder together, if necessary.
2. Salt, black pepper, and cumin are used to season the fish. In a pan, heat the oil over medium to high heat. After inserting the fillets, simmer for 3 minutes. With a spatula, rotate the fish. When weighed with a fork, cook for 3 minutes, or before the fish easily flakes. Drizzle half a teaspoon of lime juice over each serving.
3. Every fish fillet should be cut in half lengthwise to produce 8 pieces. Spoon the combination of the sour cream onto the tortillas. Fill 1 slice of fish with each tortilla. With the remaining salsa and cabbage, seal.

TIPS: If you want to add some avocado to these tacos, their buttery taste with the crunchy cabbage is perfect.

Nutrition: Calories: 385; Total Fat: 14 g; Cholesterol: 68 mg; Sodium: 1002 mg; Total Carb: 37 g; Dietary Fiber: 3 g; Sugar: 5 g; Protein: 28 g; Calcium: 12 mg; Iron: 16 mg; Potassium: 13 mg

141. Salmon with Veggies

Servings: 4
Difficulty: 1
Preparation Time: 15 minutes
Cooking Time: 6 minutes
Optavia Counts: 1 lean/ 5 green/ 1 healthy fat/ 1 condiments
Ingredients:

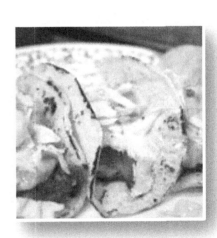

- 1 pound skin-on salmon fillets
- Salt and ground black pepper, as required
- 1 fresh parsley sprig
- 1 fresh dill sprig
- 1 tsp. coconut oil, melted and divided
- ½ lemon, sliced thinly
- 1 carrot, peeled and julienned
- 1 zucchini, peeled and julienned
- 1 red bell pepper, seeded and julienned

Directions:

1. Season the salmon fillets with salt and black pepper.
2. Arrange a steamer trivet and put herb sprigs and 1 cup of water at the bottom of the Instant Pot.
3. Place the salmon fillets, skin side down on top of the trivet.
4. Drizzle salmon fillets with 2 teaspoons of coconut oil and top with lemon slices.
5. Secure the lid and turn to the "Seal" position.
6. Choose "Steam" and use the default time of 3 minutes only.
7. Press "Cancel" and do a "Natural" release.
8. Meanwhile, for the sauce: In a bowl, add remaining ingredients and mix until well combined.
9. Remove the lid and transfer the salmon fillets onto a platter.
10. Remove the steamer trivet, herbs, and cooking water from the pot. With paper towels, pat dry the pot.
11. Place the remaining coconut oil in the Instant Pot and select "Sauté." Then add the veggies and cook for about 2–3 minutes.
12. Press "Cancel" and transfer the veggies onto a platter with salmon.

Nutrition: Calories: 204; Fat: 10.6 g; Protein: 23.1 g; Carbohydrate: 5.7 g; Net Carbohydrate: 4.3 g; Fiber: 1.4 g.

142. Lemon, Buttered Shrimp Panini

Servings: 4
Difficulty: 1
Preparation Time: 10 minutes
Cooking Time: 15 minutes
Servings: 4
Optavia Counts: 1 lean/ 5 green/ 1 healthy fat/ 4 condiments
Ingredients:

- 1 tbsp. butter
- 2 slices baguette
- 1 tsp. hot sauce
- 1 tbsp. parsley
- 1 tbsp. lemon juice
- 4 garlic cloves, minced
- 1 pound shrimp peeled

Directions:

1. Make a hollowed portion on your baguette.
2. Sauté the following on a skillet with melted butter: parsley, hot sauce, lemon juice, and garlic. After a minute or 2, mix in the shrimps and sauté for 5 minutes.
3. Scoop shrimps into baguette and grill in a Panini press until baguette is crisped and ridged.

Nutrition: Calories: 262; Carbohydrate: 14 g; Protein: 26 g; Fat: 10.8 g.

143. Baked Cod Crusted with Herbs

Servings: 4
Difficulty: 1
Preparation Time: 5 minutes
Cooking Time: 10 minutes
Optavia Counts: 1 lean/ 0 green/ 1 healthy fat/ 8 condiments
Ingredients:

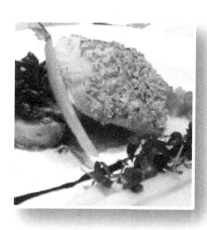

- ¼ cup honey - ¼ tsp. salt
- ½ cup panko
- ½ tsp. pepper
- 1 tbsp. extra-virgin olive oil
- 1 tbsp. lemon juice
- 1 tsp. dried basil
- 1 tsp. dried parsley
- 1 tsp. rosemary
- 4 pieces (6-8-oz.) cod fillets

Directions:

1. With olive oil, grease a 9 x 13-inch baking pan and preheat the oven to 375°F. In a Ziploc bag, mix panko, rosemary, salt, pepper, parsley, and basil. Evenly spread cod fillets in a prepped dish and drizzle with lemon juice. Then brush the fillets with honey on all sides. Discard remaining honey, if any.
2. Then evenly divide the panko mixture on top of cod fillets.
3. Pop in the oven and bake for ten minutes or until fish is cooked.

Nutrition: Calories: 137; Protein: 5 g; Fat: 2 g; Carbs: 21 g.

144. Crazy Saganaki Shrimp

Servings: 4
Difficulty: 1
Preparation Time: 10 minutes
Cooking Time: 10 minutes
Optavia Counts: 1 lean/ 1 green/ 2 healthy fat/ 6 condiments

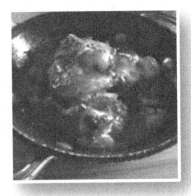

Ingredients:

- ¼ tsp. salt - ½ cup Chardonnay
- ½ cup crumbled Greek feta cheese
- 1 medium bulb. fennel, cored and finely chopped
- 1 small Chile pepper, seeded and minced
- 1 tbsp. extra-virgin olive oil
- 12 jumbo shrimps, deveined with tails left on
- 1 tbsp. lemon juice, divided
- 4 scallions sliced thinly - Pepper to taste

Directions:

1. In a medium bowl, mix salt, lemon juice, and shrimp. On medium fire, place a saganaki pan (or large non-stick saucepan) and heat oil. Sauté Chile pepper, scallions, and fennel for 4 minutes or until starting to brown and is already soft. Add wine and sauté for another minute.
2. Place shrimps on top of the fennel, cover, and cook for 4 minutes or until shrimps are pink.
3. Remove just the shrimp and transfer to a plate. Add pepper, feta, and 1 tablespoon of lemon juice to the pan and cook for a minute or until cheese begins to melt.
4. To serve, place cheese and fennel mixture on a serving plate and top with shrimps.

Nutrition: Calories: 310; Protein: 49.7 g; Fat: 6.8 g; Carbs: 8.4 g.

CHAPTER 9.

POULTRY RECIPES

145. Poppin' Pop Corn Chicken

Servings: 1
Difficulty: 1
Preparation Time: 5 minutes
Cooking Time: 15 minutes
Optavia Counts: 1 lean/ 0 green/ 0 healthy fat/ 4 condiments
Ingredients:

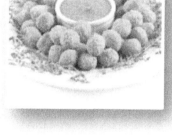

- 1 pound skinless, boneless chicken breast
- 1 tsp. chili flakes
- 1 tsp. garlic powder
- ½ cup flour
- 1 tbsp. olive oil cooking spray

Directions:

1. Preheat your fryer at 365°F. Spray with olive oil.
2. Cut the chicken breasts into cubes and place them in a bowl. Toss with the chili flakes, garlic powder, and additional seasonings to taste and make sure to coat entirely. Add the coconut flour and toss once more.
3. Cook the chicken in the fryer for ten minutes. Turnover and cook for a further five minutes before serving.

Nutrition: Calories: 383; Fat: 21 g; Carbs: 6 g; Protein: 30 g.

146. Chicken Breast with Asparagus

Servings: 1
Difficulty: 1
Preparation Time: 15 minutes
Cooking Time: 16 minutes
Optavia Counts: 1 lean/ 1 green/ 2 healthy fat/ 4 condiments
Ingredients:
For Chicken:

- ¼ cup extra-virgin olive oil
- ¼ cup fresh lemon juice
- 1 tbsp. maple syrup
- 3-4 garlic clove, minced
- Salt and ground black pepper, as required
- 4 (6-ounce) boneless, skinless chicken breasts

For Asparagus:

- 1 ½ pound fresh asparagus
- 1 tbsp. extra-virgin olive oil

Directions:

1. For the marinade: in a large bowl, add oil, lemon juice, Erythritol, garlic, salt and black pepper and beat until well combined.
2. In a large resealable plastic bag, place the chicken and ¾ cup of marinade.
3. Seal the bag and shake to coat well. Refrigerate overnight.
4. Cover the bowl of remaining marinade and refrigerate before serving.
5. Preheat the grill to medium fire. Grease the grill grate.
6. Remove the chicken from the bag and discard the marinade.
7. Place the chicken onto grill grate and grill, covered, for about 5-8 minutes per side.
8. Meanwhile, in a pan of boiling water, arrange a steamer basket.
9. Place the asparagus in a steamer basket and steam, covered, for about 5-7 minutes.
10. Drain the asparagus well and transfer it into a bowl. Add oil and toss to coat well.
11. Divide the chicken breasts and asparagus onto serving plates and serve.

Nutrition Per Serving: Calories: 319; Fat: 12.6 g; Carbs: 11 g; Fiber: 2.9 g; Sugar: 6 g; Protein: 42.3 g.

147. Chicken with Bell Peppers

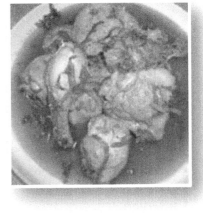

Servings: 1
Difficulty: 1
Preparation Time: 15 minutes
Cooking Time: 20 minutes
Optavia Counts: 1 lean/ 3 green/ 1 healthy fat/ 5 condiments
Ingredients:

- 1 tbsp. olive oil, divided
- 1 yellow bell pepper, seeded and sliced
- 1 red bell pepper, seeded and sliced
- 1 green bell pepper, seeded and sliced
- 1 medium onion, sliced
- 1-pound boneless, skinless chicken breasts, sliced thinly1 tsp. dried oregano, crushed
- ¼ tsp. garlic powder
- ¼ tsp. ground cumin
- Salt and freshly ground black pepper, as required
- ¼ cup low-sodium chicken broth

Directions:

1. In a wok, heat 1 tablespoon of oil over medium-high flame and cook the bell peppers and onion slices for about 4-5 minutes. With a slotted spoon, transfer the peppers mixture onto a plate.
2. In the same wok, heat the remaining oil over medium-high flame and cook the chicken for about 8 minutes, stirring frequently. Stir in the thyme, spices, salt, black pepper, and broth, and bring to a boil.
3. Add the peppers mixture and stir to combine. Reduce the heat to medium and cook for about 3-5 minutes or until all the liquid is absorbed, stirring occasionally.
4. Serve immediately.

Nutrition Per Serving: Calories: 232; Fat: 12.8 g; Carbs: 6.5 g; Fiber: 1.3 g; Sugar: 3.8 g; Protein: 22.8 g; Sodium: 98 mg.

148. Vinegar Chicken

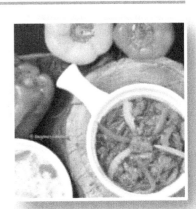

Servings: 1
Difficulty: 1
Preparation Time: 15 minutes
Cooking Time: 10 minutes
Optavia Counts: 1 lean/ 0 green/ 1 healthy fat/ 4 condiments
Ingredients:

- 1 pound chicken wings, skinless
- 1 tbsp. apple cider vinegar
- ½ tsp. salt
- ½ tsp. oregano, dried
- 1 tsp. sweet paprika
- 1 tbsp. olive oil

Directions:

1. Preheat the grill to 375°F.
2. Meanwhile, in the mixing bowl, mix up chicken wings with the vinegar and the rest of the ingredients and rub well.
3. Then put the wings in the grill and cook them for 10 minutes.
4. The cooked wings should have a golden-brown color.

Nutrition: Calories 208; Fat 14.1 g; Fiber 3.3 g; Carbs 10.5 g; Protein 18.4 g.

149. Chicken with Zoodles

Servings: 1
Difficulty: 1
Preparation Time: 15 minutes
Cooking Time: 18 minutes
Optavia Counts: 1 lean/ 1 green/ 3 healthy fat/ 8 condiments
Ingredients:

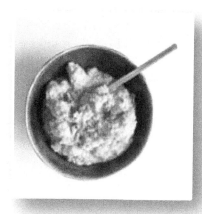

- 3 small zucchini, spiralized with Blade
- Salt, as required
- 1 ½ pounds boneless, skinless chicken breasts
- Freshly ground black pepper, as required
- 1 tbsp. olive oil
- 1 cup low-fat plain Greek yogurt
- ¼ cup low-fat Parmesan cheese, shredded
- ½ cup low-sodium chicken broth
- ½ tsp. Italian seasoning
- ½ tsp. garlic powder
- 1 cup fresh spinach, chopped
- 3-6 slices sun-dried tomatoes
- 1 tbsp. garlic, chopped

Directions:

1. Preheat your oven to 350°F. Line a large baking sheet with a parchment paper.
2. Place the zucchini noodles and salt onto the prepared baking sheet and toss to coat well.
3. Arrange the zucchini noodles in an even layer and bake for approximately 15 minutes.
4. Meanwhile, season the chicken breasts with salt and black pepper.
5. In a large wok, heat the oil over medium-high heat and cook the chicken breasts for about 4-5 minutes per side or until cooked through. With a slotted spoon, transfer the cooked chicken onto a plate and set it aside. In the same wok, add the yogurt, Parmesan cheese, broth, Italian seasoning and garlic powder and beat until well combined. Place the wok over medium-high heat and cook for about 2-3 minutes or until it starts to thicken, stirring continuously. Stir in the spinach, sun-dried tomatoes and garlic and cook for about 2-3 minutes. Add the chicken breasts and cook for about 1-2 minutes.
6. Divide the zucchini noodles onto serving plates and top each with chicken mixture. Serve immediately.

Nutrition Per Serving: Calories: 285; Fat: 7.9 g; Carbs: 8.4 g; Fiber: 1 g; Sugar: 5 g; Protein: 45.5 g; Sodium: 308 mg.

150. Chicken And Cauliflower

Servings: 2
Difficulty: 2
Preparation Time: 10 minutes
Cooking Time: 30 minutes
Optavia Counts: 1 lean/ 2 green/ 1 healthy fat/ 4 condiments
Ingredients:

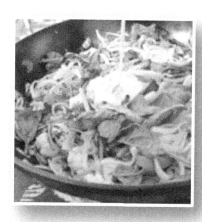

- 1 cup cauliflower florets
- ¼ carrot, chopped
- 10 oz. chicken fillet, cubed, skinless
- 1 tsp. balsamic vinegar
- 1 tbsp. olive oil
- ½ tsp. ground turmeric
- 1 tsp. minced garlic
- ½ tsp. salt

Directions:

1. Heat a pan with the oil over medium fire. Add the meat and cook for 10 minutes.
2. Add the rest of the ingredients and cook for 20 minutes more and serve.

Nutrition: Calories 276; Fat 16.4 g; Fiber 5.1 g; Carbs 13.5 g; Protein 28.4 g.

151. Chicken and Bok Choy

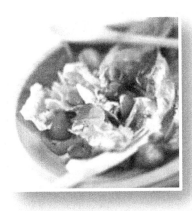

Servings: 2
Difficulty: 3
Preparation Time: 15 minutes
Cooking Time: 30 minutes
Optavia Counts: 1 lean/ 3 green/ 1 healthy fat/ 2 condiments
Ingredients:

- 1 pound chicken breast, skinless, boneless, and cubed
- 1 cup bok choy, torn
- 1 tbsp. olive oil
- ¼ tsp. minced garlic
- 1 tsp. shallots, chopped
- ½ tsp. salt
- 1 cup crushed tomatoes

Directions:

1. Heat a pan with the oil over medium-high fire. Add the chicken and cook for 10 minutes.
2. Add the rest of the ingredients and cook for 20 minutes more and serve.

Nutrition: Calories 384; Fat 32.1 g; Fiber 3 g; Carbs 6.9 g; Protein 21.6 g.

152. Chicken & Strawberry Lettuce Wraps

Servings: 2
Difficulty: 3
Preparation Time: 15 minutes
Cooking Time: 0 minutes
Optavia Counts: 1 lean/ 3 green/ 0 healthy fat/ 0 condiments
Ingredients:

- 8 oz. cooked chicken breast, cut into strips
- ½ cup fresh strawberries, hulled and sliced thinly
- ½ English cucumber, sliced thinly
- 1 tbsp. fresh mint leaves, minced
- 1 large lettuce leaves

Directions:

1. In a large bowl, add all ingredients except lettuce leaves and gently toss to coat well.
2. Place the lettuce leaves onto serving plates.
3. Place the chicken mixture over each lettuce leaf evenly and serve immediately.

Nutrition Per Serving: Calories: 165; Fat: 2.9 g; Carbs: 8.8 g; Fiber: 1.7 g; Sugar: 4.4 g; Protein: 26 g; Sodium: 58 mg.

153. Orange Chicken

Servings: 2
Difficulty: 1
Preparation Time: 10 minutes
Cooking Time: 20 minutes
Optavia Counts: 1 lean/ 1 green/ 0 healthy fat/ 7 condiments
Ingredients:

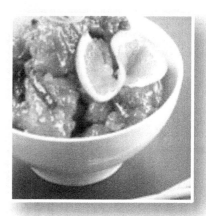

- 2 garlic cloves, minced
- ½ cup fresh orange juice
- 1 tbsp. apple cider vinegar
- 1 tbsp. low-sodium soy sauce
- ¼ tsp. ground ginger
- ¼ tsp. ground cinnamon
- Freshly ground black pepper, as required
- 8 skinless, bone-in chicken thighs
- ⅓ cup scallion, sliced

Directions:

1. To marinate in a large bowl, mix together all ingredients except for chicken thighs and scallion.
2. Add the chicken thighs and coat with marinade generously.
3. Cover the bowl and refrigerate to marinate for about 4 hours.
4. Remove the chicken from the bowl, reserving marinade.
5. Heat a lightly greased large non-stick wok over medium-high fire and cook the chicken thighs for about 5-6 minutes or till golden brown.
6. Flip the side and cook for about 4 minutes.
7. Stir in the reserved marinade and bring to a boil.
8. Reduce the heat to medium-low and cook, covered for about 6-8 minutes or until sauce becomes thick.
9. Stir in the scallion and remove from the heat.
10. Serve hot.

Nutrition Per Serving: Calories: 205; Fat: 5.5 g; Carbs: 3.6 g; Fiber: 0.3 g; Sugar: 2.2 g; Protein: 34.4 g; Sodium: 349 mg.

154. Chicken Stuffed Avocado

Servings: 2
Difficulty: 3
Preparation Time: 15 minutes
Cooking Time: 0 minutes
Optavia Counts: 1 lean/ 0 green/ 2 healthy fat/ 4 condiments
Ingredients:

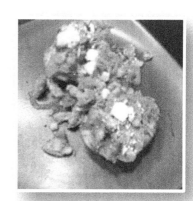

- 1 cup cooked chicken, shredded
- 1 avocado, halved and pitted
- 1 tbsp. fresh lime juice
- ¼ cup yellow onion, chopped finely
- ¼ cup low-fat plain Greek yogurt
- Pinch of cayenne pepper
- Salt and ground black pepper, as required

Directions:

1. With a small scooper, scoop out the flesh from the middle of each avocado half and transfer it into a bowl.
2. In the bowl of avocado flesh, add the lime juice and with a fork, mash until well blended.
3. Add remaining ingredients and stir to combine.
4. Divide the chicken mixture into avocado halves evenly and serve immediately.

Nutrition Per Serving: Calories: 281; Fat: 15 g; Carbs: 9 g; Fiber: 5 g; Sugar: 3.2 g; Protein: 23.7 g; Sodium: 176 mg.

155. Chicken & Veggies Stir Fry

Servings: 3
Difficulty: 1
Preparation Time: 15 minutes
Cooking Time: 15 minutes
Optavia Counts: 1 lean/ 2 green/ 2 healthy fat/ 7 condiments
Ingredients:

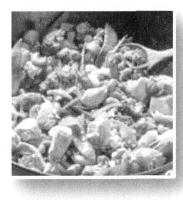

- 1 tbsp. fresh lime juice
- 1 tbsp. fish sauce
- 1 ½ tsp. arrowroot starch
- 1 tsp. olive oil, divided
- 1-pound skinless, boneless chicken tenders, cubed
- 1 tsp. fresh ginger, minced
- 2 garlic cloves, minced
- ¾ tsp. red pepper flakes, crushed
- ¼ cup water
- 2 cups broccoli, cut into bite-sized pieces
- 2 cups red bell pepper, seeded and sliced
- ¼ cup pine nuts

Directions:

1. In a bowl, add lime juice, fish sauce, and arrowroot starch and mix until well combined. Set aside.
2. In a large non-stick sauté pan, heat 2 teaspoons of oil over high flame and cook chicken for about 6-8 minutes, stirring frequently.
3. Transfer the chicken into a bowl and set it aside.
4. In the same sauté pan, heat remaining oil over medium flame and sauté ginger, garlic and red pepper flakes for about 1 minute.
5. Add water, broccoli and bell pepper and stir fry for about 2-3 minutes.
6. Stir in chicken and lime juice mixture and cook for about 2-3 minutes.
7. Stir in pine nuts and immediately remove from heat.
8. Serve hot.

Nutrition Per Serving: Calories: 207; Fat: 10.7 g; Carbs: 10 g; Fiber: 2.7 g; Sugar: 4.5 g; Protein: 20.4 g; Sodium: 513 mg.

156. Chicken & Broccoli Bake

Servings: 3
Difficulty: 2
Preparation Time: 15 minutes
Cooking Time: 24 minutes
Optavia Counts: 1 lean/ 1 green/ 2 healthy fat/ 4 condiments
Ingredients:

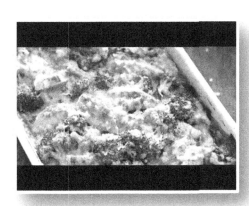

- Olive oil cooking spray
- 1/14 pounds (6-ounce) skinless, boneless chicken thighs
- 2 broccoli heads, cut into florets
- 1 garlic cloves, minced
- ¼ cup extra-virgin olive oil
- 1 tsp. dried oregano, crushed
- 1 tsp. dried rosemary, crushed
- Salt and freshly ground black pepper, as required

Directions:

1. Preheat your oven to 375°F.
2. Grease a large baking dish with cooking spray.
3. In a large bowl, add all the ingredients and toss to coat well.
4. In the bottom of the prepared baking dish, arrange the broccoli florets and top with chicken breasts in a single layer.
5. Bake for approximately 45 minutes.
6. Serve hot.

Nutrition Per Serving: Calories: 333; Fat: 15 g; Carbs: 9.4 g; Fiber: 3.6 g; Sugar: 2.2 g; Protein: 41.7 g; Sodium: 130 mg.

157. Cheesy Chicken & Spinach

Servings: 3
Difficulty: 1
Preparation Time: 15 minutes
Cooking Time: 20 minutes
Optavia Counts: 1 lean/ 1 green/ 2 healthy fat/ 4 condiments

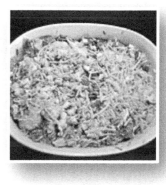

Ingredients:
- 1 tbsp. olive oil, divided
- 6 boneless, skinless chicken thighs (about 1-1/2 pounds)
- Salt and ground black pepper, as required
- 2 garlic cloves, minced
- 2 jalapeño pepper, chopped
- 10-oz. frozen spinach, thawed
- ⅓ cup low-fat Parmesan cheese, shredded

Directions:
1. In a large wok, heat 1 tablespoon of the oil over medium-high flame and cook the chicken with salt and black pepper for about 5-6 minutes per side.
2. Transfer the chicken into a bowl.
3. In the same wok, heat the remaining oil over medium-low fire and sauté the garlic for about 1 minute.
4. Add the spinach and cook for about 1 minute.
5. Add the cheese, salt and black pepper and stir to combine.
6. Spread the spinach mixture in the bottom of the wok evenly.
7. Place chicken over spinach in a single layer.
8. Immediately adjust the heat to low and cook, covered for about 5 minutes.
9. Serve hot.

Nutrition Per Serving: Calories: 323; Fat: 17.5 g; Carbs: 3.5 g; Fiber: 1.7 g; Sugar: 0.4gProtein: 37.5 g; Sodium: 267 mg.

158. Chicken with Mushrooms

Servings: 3
Difficulty: 1
Preparation Time: 15 minutes
Cooking Time: 20 minutes
Optavia Counts: 1 lean/ 1 green/ 2 healthy fat/ 6 condiments

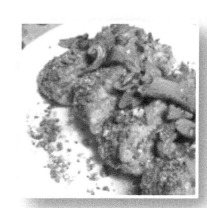

Ingredients:
- 1 tbsp. almond flour
- Salt and freshly ground black pepper, as required
- 6 (4-ounce) skinless, boneless chicken breasts
- 1 tbsp. olive oil
- 3 garlic cloves, chopped
- ¾ pound fresh mushrooms, sliced
- ¾ cup low-sodium chicken broth
- ¼ cup balsamic vinegar
- 2 bay leaf
- ¼ tsp. dried thyme

Directions:
1. In a bowl, mix together the flour, salt and black pepper.
2. Coat the chicken breasts with flour mixture evenly.
3. In a wok, heat the olive oil over medium-high heat and stir fry the chicken for about 3 minutes.
4. Add the garlic and flip the chicken breasts. Spread mushrooms over chicken and cook for about 3 minutes, shaking the wok frequently. Add the broth, vinegar, bay leaf and thyme and stir to combine.
5. Reduce the heat to medium-low and simmer, covered for about 10 minutes, flipping chicken occasionally. With a slotted spoon, transfer the chicken onto a warm serving platter and with a piece of foil, cover to keep warm. Place the pan of sauce over medium-high heat and cook, uncovered, for about 7 minutes. Remove the pan from heat and discard the bay leaf.
6. Place mushroom sauce over chicken and serve hot.

Nutrition Per Serving: Calories: 247; Fat: 11.4 g; Carbs: 7.6 g; Fiber: 1.1 g; Sugar: 1.6 g; Protein: 29.1 g; Sodium: 99 mg.

159. Whole Chicken Roast

Servings: 3
Difficulty: 4
Preparation Time: 15 minutes
Cooking Time: 90 minutes
Optavia Counts: 1 lean/ 0 green/ 1 healthy fat/ 4 condiments
Ingredients:

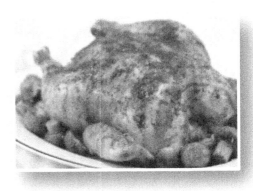

- 3-pound whole chicken, skinless, lean
- 1 tbsp. sweet paprika
- 1 lemon juice
- 1 tbsp. avocado oil
- 1 tsp. salt
- 1 tsp. chili powder

Directions:

1. Rub the chicken with lemon juice, paprika, oil, salt, and chili powder. Transfer it to the tray.
2. Bake the chicken for 90 min at 365°F.

Nutrition: Calories: 359; Fat: 13.5 g; Fiber: 4.9 g; Carbs: 17.6 g; Protein: 49.7 g.

160. Basil Duck Fillet

Servings: 4
Difficulty: 1
Preparation Time: 10 minutes
Cooking Time: 15 minutes
Optavia Counts: 1 lean/ 0 green/ 1 healthy fat/ 5 condiments
Ingredients:

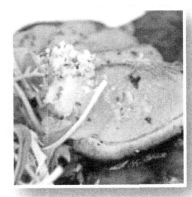

- Juice of 1 lime
- 1 tbsp. dried basil
- ½ tsp. ground black pepper
- 1 tsp. salt
- 1 tsp. sweet paprika
- ⅓ cup water
- 2 pounds' duck fillets, skinless
- 1 tsp. olive oil

Directions:

1. Heat a pan with the oil over medium fire; add the duck fillets and cook for 5 minutes.
2. Add the rest of the ingredients and cook the duck legs for 10 minutes with the closed lid.

Nutrition: Calories: 142; Fat: 4.8 g; Fiber: 3.6 g; Carbs: 11.7 g; Protein: 22.1 g.

161. Chicken with Broccoli & Mushrooms

Servings: 4
Difficulty: 2
Preparation Time: 15 minutes
Cooking Time: 22 minutes
Optavia Counts: 1 lean/ 2 green/ 1 healthy fat/ 5 condiments
Ingredients:

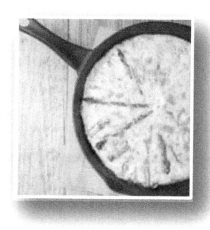

- 1 tbsp. olive oil, divided
- 4 boneless, skinless chicken breasts, cut into small pieces
- Salt and freshly ground black pepper, as required
- 1 onion, chopped finely
- 1 tsp. fresh ginger, grated
- 1 tsp. garlic, minced
- 1 cup broccoli florets
- 1 ½ cups fresh mushrooms, sliced
- ¼ cup low-sodium chicken broth

Directions:

1. In a large wok, heat 1 tablespoon of oil over medium-high heat and stir fry the chicken pieces, salt, and black pepper for about 4-5 minutes or until golden brown.
2. With a slotted spoon, transfer the chicken onto a plate.
3. In the same wok, heat the remaining oil over medium-high heat and sauté the onion, ginger, and garlic for about 4-5 minutes.
4. Add in mushrooms and cook for about 4-5 minutes, stirring frequently.
5. Add the broccoli and stir fry for about 3 minutes.
6. Add the cooked chicken and broth and stir fry for about 3-5 minutes.
7. Add in the salt and black pepper and remove from the heat.
8. Serve hot.

Nutrition Per Serving: Calories: 211; Fat: 8.7 g; Carbs: 5.7 g; Fiber: 1.5 g; Sugar: 2 g; Protein: 28.4 g; Sodium: 1141 mg.

162. Chicken & Asparagus Frittata

Servings: 4
Difficulty: 2
Preparation Time: 15 minutes
Cooking Time: 12 minutes
Optavia Counts: 2 lean/ 2 green/ 2 healthy fat/ 1 condiments
Ingredients:

- ½ cup cooked chicken, chopped
- ⅓ cup low-fat Parmesan cheese, grated
- 2 eggs, beaten lightly
- Salt and ground black pepper, as required
- 1 tsp. coconut oil
- ½ cup boiled asparagus, chopped
- 1 tbsp. fresh parsley, chopped

Directions:

1. Preheat the broiler of the oven.
2. In a bowl, add the cheese, eggs, salt and black pepper and beat until well combined.
3. In a large ovenproof wok, melt coconut oil over medium-high heat and cook the chicken and asparagus for about 2-3 minutes. Add the egg mixture and stir to combine.Cook for about 4-5 minutes.
4. Remove from the heat and sprinkle with the parsley.
5. Now, transfer the wok under the broiler and broil for about 3-4 minutes or until slightly puffed.
6. Cut into desired-sized wedges and serve immediately.

Nutrition Per Serving: Calories: 156; Fat: 9.9 g; Carbs: 1.3 g; Fiber: 0.4 g; Sugar: 0.8 g; Protein: 15.4 g; Sodium: 270 mg.

163. Chicken & Zucchini Muffins

Servings: 4
Difficulty: 2
Preparation Time: 15 minutes
Cooking Time: 15 minutes
Optavia Counts: 2 lean/ 2 green/ 5 healthy fat/ 2 condiments
Ingredients:

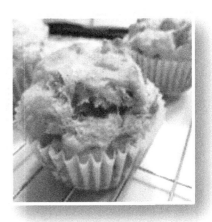

- 4 eggs
- ¼ cup olive oil
- ¼ cup water
- ⅓ cup coconut flour
- ½ tsp. baking powder
- ¼ tsp. salt
- ¾ cup cooked chicken, shredded
- ¾ cup zucchini, grated
- ½ cup low-fat Parmesan cheese, shredded
- 1 tbsp. fresh oregano, minced
- 1 tbsp. fresh thyme, minced
- ¼ cup low-fat cheddar cheese, grated

Directions:

1. Preheat your oven to 400°F.
2. Lightly grease 8 cups of a muffin pan.
3. In a bowl, add eggs, oil and water and beat until well combined.
4. Add the flour, baking powder, and salt, and mix well.
5. Add the remaining ingredients and mix until just combined.
6. Place the muffin mixture into the prepared muffin cup evenly.
7. Bake for approximately 13-15 minutes or until the tops become golden brown.
8. Remove muffin pan from oven and place onto a wire rack to cool for about 10 minutes.
9. Invert the muffins onto a platter and serve warm.

Nutrition Per Serving: Calories: 321; Fat: 24.2 g; Carbs: 8.1 g; Fiber: 4.3 g; Sugar: 1.5 g; Protein: 19.2 g; Sodium: 484 mg.

164. Chicken & Bell Pepper Muffins

Servings: 4
Difficulty: 2
Preparation Time: 15 minutes
Cooking Time: 20 minutes
Optavia Counts: 2 lean/ 1 green/ 0 healthy fat/ 2 condiments
Ingredients:

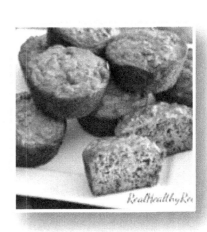

- 2 eggs
- Salt and ground black pepper, as required
- 1 tbsp. water
- 8 oz. cooked chicken, chopped finely
- 1 cup green bell pepper, seeded and chopped
- 1 cup onion, chopped

Directions:

1. Preheat your oven to 350°F.
2. Grease 8 cups of a muffin tin.
3. In a bowl, add eggs, black pepper and water and beat until well combined.
4. Add the chicken, bell pepper and onion and stir to combine.
5. Transfer the mixture to prepared muffin cups evenly.
6. Bake for approximately 18-20 minutes or until golden brown.
7. Remove the muffin tin from the oven and place it onto a wire rack to cool for about 10 minutes.
8. Carefully invert the muffins onto a platter and serve warm.

Nutrition Per Serving: Calories: 232; Fat: 10.6 g; Carbs: 5.6 g; Fiber: 1 g; Sugar: 3.4 g; Protein: 28.1 g; Sodium: 161 mg.

165. Chicken Stroganoff

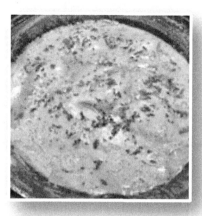

Servings: 4
Difficulty: 2
Preparation Time: 10 minutes
Cooking Time: 20 minutes
Optavia Counts: 1 lean/ 1 green/ 2 healthy fat/ 3 condiments
Ingredients:

- 1 cup cremini mushrooms, sliced
- 1 onion, sliced
- 1 tbsp. olive oil
- ½ tsp. thyme
- 1 tsp. salt
- 1 cup Plain yogurt
- 10 oz. chicken fillet, chopped

Directions:

1. Heat up olive oil in the saucepan.
2. Add mushrooms and onion.
3. Sprinkle the vegetables with thyme and salt. Mix up well and cook them for 5 minutes.
4. After this, add chopped chicken fillet and mix up well.
5. Cook the ingredients for 5 minutes more.
6. Then add plain yogurt, mix up well, and close the lid.
7. Cook chicken stroganoff for 10 minutes over low heat.

Nutrition: Calories 224; Fat 9.2 g; Fiber 0.8 g; Carbs 7.4 g; Protein 24.2 g.

CHAPTER 10.

VEGAN & VEGETARIAN RECIPES

166. Quinoa Porridge

Serving: 1
Difficulty: 1
Preparation Time: 5 minutes
Cooking Time: 25 minutes
Optavia Counts: 0 lean/ 0 green/ 1 healthy fat/ 1 condiments
Ingredients:

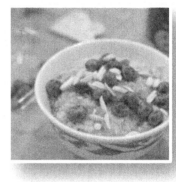

- ¾ cups coconut milk
- 1 cup rinsed quinoa
- ⅛ tsp. ground cinnamon
- 1 cup fresh blueberries

Directions:

1. In a saucepan, boil the coconut milk over high heat. Add the quinoa to the milk then bring the mixture to a boil.
2. Let it simmer for 15 minutes on medium heat until the milk is reduced. Add the cinnamon and mix it properly in the saucepan.
3. Cover the saucepan and cook for at least 8 minutes until the milk is completely absorbed.
4. Add in the blueberries and cook for 30 more seconds. Serve.

Nutrition: Calories: 271; Fat: 3.7 g; Carbs: 54 g; Protein: 6.5 g.

167. Potato Hash with Cilantro-Lime Cream

Serving: 1
Difficulty: 2
Preparation Time: 20 minutes
Cooking Time: 30 minutes
Optavia Counts: 0 lean/ 3 green/ 3 healthy fat/ 11 condiments
Ingredients:
For the Cilantro-Lime Cream:

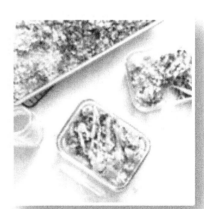

- 4 avocado, halved and pitted
- ¼ cup packed fresh cilantro leaves and stems
- 1 tbsp. freshly squeezed lime juice
- 1 garlic clove, peeled
- 1 tsp. kosher salt
- ½ tsp. ground cumin
- 1 tbsp. extra-virgin olive oil

For the Hash:

- ½ tsp. kosher salt
- 1 large sweet potato, cut into ¾-inch pieces
- 2 tbsp. extra-virgin olive oil
- 1 onion, thinly sliced
- 2 garlic cloves, crushed
- 1 red bell pepper, thinly sliced
- 1 tsp. ground cumin
- ¼ tsp. ground turmeric
- A pinch of freshly ground black pepper
- 2 tbsp. fresh cilantro leaves, chopped
- ½ jalapeño pepper, seeded and chopped (optional)
- Hot sauce, for serving (optional)

Directions:

To Make the Cilantro-Lime Cream:

1. Add the avocado flesh to a food compressor. Add the cilantro, lime juice, garlic, salt, and cumin. Whirl until smooth. Taste and adjust seasonings, as needed. If you do not have a food processor or blender, simply mash the avocado well with a fork; the results will have more texture, but will still work. Cover and refrigerate until ready to serve.

To Make the Hash:

2. Boil salt water in a medium pot over high heat. Add the sweet potato and cook for about 20 minutes until tender. Drain thoroughly.
3. Heat olive oil in a big skillet over low fire until it shimmers. Add the onion and sauté for about 4 minutes until translucent. Put the garlic and cook, turning, for about 30 seconds. Add the cooked sweet potato and red bell pepper. Season the hash with cumin, salt, turmeric, and pepper. Sauté for 5 to 7 minutes, until the sweet potatoes are golden and the red bell pepper is soft.
4. Divide the sweet potatoes between 2 bowls and spoon the sauce over them. Scatter the cilantro and jalapeño (optional) over each and serve with hot sauce (optional).

Nutrition: Calories: 520; Total fat: 43 g; Cholesterol: 0 mg; Fiber: 2 g; Protein: 12 g; Sodium: 1719 mg.

168. Millet Porridge

Serving: 1
Difficulty: 2
Preparation Time: 10 minutes
Cooking Time: 20 minutes
Optavia Counts: 0 lean/ 0 green/ 1 healthy fat/ 4 condiments
Ingredients:

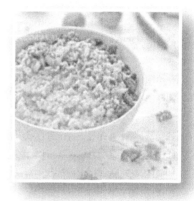

- Sea salt
- 1 tbsp. finely chopped coconuts
- ½ cup unsweetened coconut milk
- ½ cup rinsed and drained millet
- 1-½ cups alkaline water
- 12-15 drops liquid stevia

Directions:

1. Sauté the millet in a non-stick skillet for about 3 minutes. Add salt and water then stir.
2. Let the meal boil then reduce the amount of heat.
3. Cook for 15 minutes; then add the remaining ingredients. Stir. Cook the meal for 4 extra minutes.
4. Serve the meal with a topping of chopped nuts.

Nutrition: Calories: 219; Fat: 4.5 g; Carbs: 38.2 g; Protein: 6.4 g.

169. Crunchy Quinoa Meal

Serving: 2
Difficulty: 1
Preparation Time: 5 minutes
Cooking Time: 25 minutes
Optavia Counts: 0 lean/ 0 green/ 2 healthy fat/ 1 condiments
Ingredients:

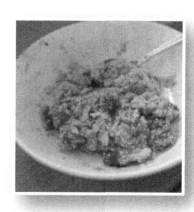

- 1 15-oz. can coconut milk
- 1 cup rinsed quinoa
- ⅛ tsp. ground cinnamon
- 1 cup raspberry
- ½ cup chopped coconuts

Directions:

1. In a saucepan, pour milk and bring it to a boil over moderate heat.
2. Add the quinoa to the milk and then bring it to a boil once more.
3. Let it simmer for at least 15 minutes on medium heat until the milk is reduced.
4. Stir in the cinnamon then mix properly.
5. Cover and cook for 8 minutes until the milk is completely absorbed.
6. Add the raspberry and cook the meal for 30 seconds. Serve and enjoy.

Nutrition: Calories: 271; Fat: 3.7 g; Carbs: 54 g; Proteins: 6.5 g.

170. Banana Barley Porridge

Serving: 2
Difficulty: 1
Preparation Time: 15 minutes
Cooking Time: 5 minutes
Optavia Counts: 0 lean/ 0 green/ 1 healthy fat/ 2 condiments
Ingredients:

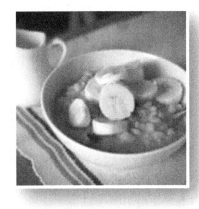

- 1 cup divided unsweetened coconut milk
- 1 small peeled and sliced banana
- ½ cup barley
- 3 drops liquid stevia
- ¼ cup chopped coconuts

Directions:

1. In a bowl, properly mix barley with half of the coconut milk and stevia.
2. Cover the mixing bowl then refrigerate for about 6 hours.
3. In a saucepan, mix the barley mixture with coconut milk. Cook for about 5 minutes on moderate heat.
4. Then top it with the chopped coconuts and the banana slices. Serve.

Nutrition: Calories: 159; Fat: 8.4 g; Carbs: 19.8 g; Proteins: 4.6 g.

171. Pumpkin Spice Quinoa

Serving: 2
Difficulty: 1
Preparation Time: 10 minutes
Cooking Time: 0 minutes
Optavia Counts: 0 lean/ 0 green/ 1 healthy fat/ 3 condiments
Ingredients:

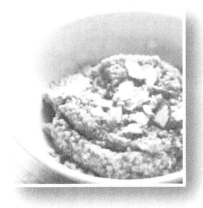

- 1 cup cooked quinoa
- 1 cup unsweetened coconut milk
- 1 large mashed banana
- ¼ cup pumpkin puree
- 1 tsp. pumpkin spice
- 1 tsp. chia seeds

Directions:

1. In a container, mix all the ingredients. Seal the lid then shake the container properly to mix.
2. Refrigerate overnight. Serve.

Nutrition: Calories: 212; Fat: 11.9 g; Carbs: 31.7 g; Protein: 7.3 g.

172. Baked Cheesy Eggplant with Marinara

Serving: 2
Difficulty: 3
Preparation Time: 20 minutes
Cooking Time: 45 minutes
Optavia Counts: 0 lean/ 1 green/ 4 healthy fat/ 6 condiments
Ingredients:

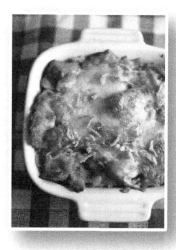

- 1 garlic clove, sliced
- 1 large eggplant
- 1 tbsp. olive oil
- ½ pinch salt, or as needed
- ¼ cup and 2 tbsp. dry breadcrumbs
- ¼ cup and 2 tbsp. vegan ricotta cheese
- ¼ cup grated vegan Parmesan cheese
- ¼ cup water, plus more as needed
- ¼ tsp. red pepper flakes
- 1 ½ cups prepared marinara sauce
- 1 1tbsp. shredded vegan pepper jack cheese
- Salt and freshly ground black pepper to taste

Directions:

1. Cut the eggplant crosswise into 5 pieces.
2. Lightly, grease skillet with 1 tablespoon of olive oil and add garlic. Heat the oil at 390°F and cook for one minute. Lower the heat to 330°F. Add the aubergines, season with pepper flakes and salt. and cook for 2 minutes on each side. Transfer to a plate. In the same skillet, stir in water and marinara sauce. Cook for 7 minutes until heated through. Stirring now and then. Transfer to a bowl.
3. In a bowl, whisk well pepper, salt, pepper jack cheese, Parmesan cheese, and ricotta. Evenly spread cheeses over eggplant strips. Lay eggplant in baking pan. Pour the marinara sauce on top.
4. In a small bowl, whisk well olive oil, and breadcrumbs. Sprinkle all over the sauce.
5. Cook for 15 minutes at 390ºF until tops are lightly browned. Serve and enjoy.

Nutrition: Calories: 405; Carbs: 41.1 g; Protein: 12.7 g; Fat: 21.4 g.

173. Baby Corn in Chili-Turmeric Spice

Serving: 2
Difficulty: 1
Preparation Time: 5 minutes
Cooking Time: 8 minutes
Optavia Counts: 0 lean/ 1 green/ 0 healthy fat/ 6 condiments
Ingredients:

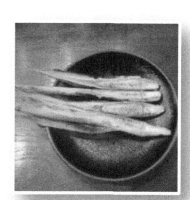

- ¼ cup water
- ¼ tsp. baking soda
- ¼ tsp. salt
- ¼ tsp. turmeric powder
- ½ tsp. curry powder
- ½ tsp. red chili powder
- 1 cup chickpea flour or bean
- 10 pieces baby corn, blanched

Directions:

1. Preheat the Air Fryer to 400ºF.
2. Line the Air Fryer basket with aluminum foil and brush with oil.
3. In a mixing bowl, mix all ingredients except for the corn.
4. Whisk until well combined.
5. Dip the corn in the batter and place it inside the Air Fryer. Cook for 8 minutes until golden brown.

Nutrition: Calories: 89; Carbs: 14.35 g; Protein: 4.75 g; Fat: 1.54 g.

174. Jackfruit Vegetable Fry

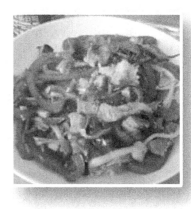

Serving: 2
Difficulty: 1
Preparation Time: 5 minutes
Cooking Time: 5 minutes
Optavia Counts: 0 lean/ 3 green/ 1 healthy fat/ 4 condiments
Ingredients:

- 4 cups finely chopped small onions
- 3 medium sized finely chopped cherry tomatoes
- ⅛ tsp. ground turmeric
- 1 tbsp. olive oil
- 1 large seeded and chopped red bell peppers
- 2 cups seeded and chopped firm jackfruit
- ⅛ tsp. cayenne pepper
- 1 tbsp. chopped fresh basil leaves
- Salt

Directions:

1. In a greased skillet, sauté the onions and bell peppers for about 5 minutes.
2. Add the tomatoes and stir. Cook for 2 minutes.
3. Then add the jackfruit, cayenne pepper, salt, and turmeric up. Cook for about 8 minutes.
4. Garnish the meal with basil leaves. Serve warm.

Nutrition: Calories: 236; Fat: 1.8 g; Carbs: 48.3 g; Protein: 7 g.

175. Zucchini Noodles with Creamy Avocado Pesto

Serving: 3
Difficulty: 1
Preparation Time: 5 minutes
Cooking Time: 20 minutes
Optavia Counts: 0 lean/ 2 green/ 3 healthy fat/ 3 condiments
Ingredients:

- 6 cups spiralized zucchini
- 1 tbsp. olive oil
- 6 oz. avocado
- 1 basil leaf
- 1 garlic cloves
- ⅓ oz. pine nuts
- 1 tbsp. lemon juice
- ½ tsp. salt
- ¼ tsp. black pepper

Directions:

1. Spiralize the courgettes and set them aside on paper towels to absorb the excess water.
2. In a food processor, put avocados, lemon juice, basil leaves, garlic, pine nuts, and sea salt and pulse until chopped.
3. Then put olive oil in a slow stream till emulsified and creamy. Drizzle olive oil in a skillet over medium-high heat and put zucchini noodles, cooking for about 2 minutes till tender.
4. Put zucchini noodles in a big bowl and toss with avocado pesto.
5. Season with cracked pepper and a little Parmesan and serve.

Nutrition: Calories: 362; Carbs: 16 g; Protein: 4.6 g; Fat: 34.1 g; Sodium: 28 mg; Potassium: 1043 mg; Fiber: 9.1 g; Sugar: 4.1 g; Calcium: 40 mg.

176. Celeriac Stuffed Avocado

Serving: 3
Difficulty: 1
Preparation Time: 10 minutes
Cooking Time: 0 minutes
Optavia Counts: 0 lean/ 0 green/ 3 healthy fat/ 3 condiments
Ingredients:

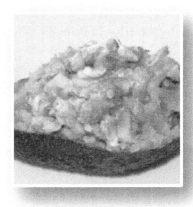

- 2 large avocado
- 1 celery root, finely chopped
- 1 tbsp. mayonnaise
- ½ of a lemon, juiced, zested
- ¼ tsp. salt

Directions:

1. Prepare avocado and for this, cut avocado in half and then remove its pit.
2. Place remaining ingredients in a bowl, stir well until combined, and evenly stuff this mixture into avocado halves. Serve.

Nutrition: Calories 285; Fats 27 g; Protein 2.8 g; Net Carb 4.4 g; Fiber 2.6 g.

177. Baked Potato Topped with Cream Cheese and Olives

Serving: 4
Difficulty: 3
Preparation Time: 15 minutes
Cooking Time: 40 minutes
Optavia Counts: 0 lean/ 2 green/ 3 healthy fat/ 3 condiments
Ingredients:

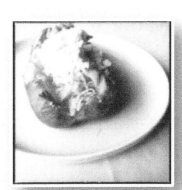

- ¼ tsp. onion powder
- 1 medium russet potato, scrubbed and peeled
- 1 tbsp. chives, chopped
- 1 tbsp. Kalamata olives
- 1 tsp. olive oil - ⅛ tsp. salt
- A dollop of vegan butter
- A dollop of vegan cream cheese

Directions:

1. Place inside the Air Fryer basket and cook for 40 minutes. Be sure to turn the potatoes once halfway through. Place the potatoes in a mixing bowl and pour in olive oil, onion powder, salt, and vegan butter.
2. Preheat the Air Fryer to 400°F. Serve the potatoes with vegan cream cheese, Kalamata olives, chives, and other vegan toppings that you want.

Nutrition: Calories: 504; Carbs: 68.34 g; Protein: 9.31 g; Fat: 21.53 g.

178. Peanut Sauce, Green Vegetables and Tempeh

Serving: 3
Difficulty: 1
Preparation Time: 25 minutes
Cooking Time: 5 minutes
Optavia Counts: 0 lean/ 4 green/ 1 healthy fat/ 6 condiments
Ingredients:
Veggies:

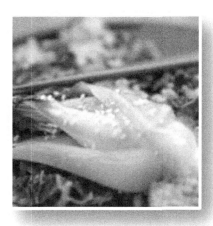

- 8 oz. tempeh, cubed
- ½ cup frozen spinach
- ½ cup green bell pepper, chopped
- ½ cup broccoli
- ¼ cup yellow onion, chopped
- ½ cup unshelled edamame
- ¼ cup vegetable broth, low-sodium
- ¼ clove minced garlic

Sauce:

- 1 tbsp. unsalted peanut butter
- 1 tbsp. soy sauce, low-sodium
- 1 tbsp. apple cider vinegar
- ¼ tsp. garlic powder

Directions:

1. Pour vegetable broth into a saucepan at low pressure.
2. In the sauce, add tempeh, bell pepper, spinach, cabbage, broccoli, edamame, along with garlic, and simmer until the vegetables are tender and the vegetable broth is soaked in.
3. Whisk all sauce ingredients together in a separate bowl while the vegetables and tempeh are cooking; if needed, add a little water for a thinner consistency.
4. Place aside sauce. If vegetables are ready to cook, apply the peanut sauce and cover uniformly.

Nutrition: Calories: 441 kcal; Carbohydrates: 43.3 g; Protein: 21.2 g; Fats: 23.7 g.

179. Spicy Waffle with Jalapeno

Serving: 3
Difficulty: 1
Preparation Time: 5 minutes
Cooking Time: 10 minutes
Optavia Counts: 1 lean/ 0 green/ 3 healthy fat/ 3 condiments
Ingredients:

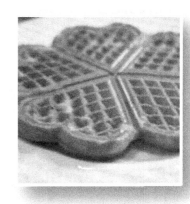

- 1 tsp. coconut flour
- ½ tbsp. chopped jalapeno pepper
- 1 tsp. cream cheese
- 2 large egg
- ½ cup shredded mozzarella cheese
- ¼ tsp. salt
- ⅛ tsp. ground black pepper

Directions:

1. Switch on a mini waffle maker and let it preheat for 5 minutes.
2. Meanwhile, take a medium bowl, place all the ingredients in it and then mix by using an immersion blender until smooth.
3. Ladle the batter evenly into the waffle maker. Shut with lid, and let it cook for 3 to 4 minutes until firm and golden brown. Serve.

Nutrition: Calories: 153; Fats: 10.7 g; Protein: 11.1 g; Net Carb: 1 g; Fiber: 1 g.

180. Green Pea Guacamole

Serving: 3
Difficulty: 2
Preparation Time: 15 minutes
Cooking Time: 35 minutes
Optavia Counts: 0 lean/ 2 green/ 0 healthy fat/ 5 condiments
Ingredients:

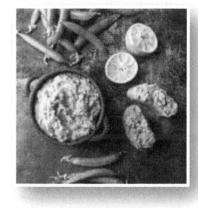

- 1 tsp. crushed garlic
- 1 chopped tomato
- 2 cups frozen green peas (chopped)
- ½ cup green onions, chopped
- 1/6 tsp. hot sauce
- ½ tsp. grounded cumin
- ½ cup lime juice

Directions:

1. Blend the peas, garlic, lime juice and cumin until it is smoothened
2. Stir in the tomatoes, green onion and hot sauce into the mixture. Then add salt to taste
3. Cover it and put it into the refrigerator for a minimum of 30 minutes.
4. This will allow the flavor to blend very well.

Nutrition: Calories: 40.7; Fat: 0.2 g; Cholesterol: 0 mg; Sodium: 157.4 mg; Carbs: 7.6g; Dietary Fiber: 1.7 g; Protein: 2.7 g.

181. Hemp Seed Porridge

Serving: 4
Difficulty: 1
Preparation Time: 5 minutes
Cooking Time: 5 minutes
Optavia Counts: 0 lean/ 0 green/ 1 healthy fat/ 2 condiments
Ingredients:

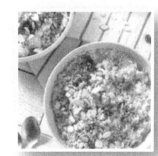

- ¼ cup cooked hemp seed
- 3 drops Stevia
- 1 cup coconut milk

Directions:

1. In a saucepan, mix the rice and the coconut milk over moderate heat for about 5 minutes as you stir it constantly.
2. Remove the pan from the burner then add the Stevia. Stir.
3. Serve in 6 bowls. Enjoy.

Nutrition: Calories: 236; Fat: 1.8 g; Carbs: 48.3 g; Protein: 7 g.

182. Coconut Pancakes

Serving: 4
Difficulty: 1
Preparation Time: 5 minutes
Cooking Time: 15 minutes
Optavia Counts: 0 lean/ 0 green/ 3 healthy fat/ 1 condiments
Ingredients:

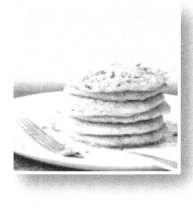

- 1 cup coconut flour
- 1 tbsp. arrowroot powder
- 1 tsp. baking powder
- 1 cup coconut milk
- 1 tbsp. coconut oil

Directions:

1. In a medium container, mix in all the dry ingredients.
2. Add the coconut milk and 2 tablespoon of coconut oil; then mix properly.
3. In a skillet, melt 1 teaspoon of coconut oil.
4. Pour a ladle of the batter into the skillet; then swirl the pan to spread the batter evenly into a smooth pancake.
5. Cook it for around 3 minutes on medium heat, until it becomes firm.
6. Turn the pancake to the other side and cook it for another 2 minutes until it turns golden brown.
7. Cook the remaining pancakes in the same manner. Serve.

Nutrition: Calories: 377; Fat: 14.9 g; Carbs: 60.7 g; Protein: 6.4 g.

183. Veggie Fritters

Serving: 4
Difficulty: 1
Preparation Time: 10 minutes
Cooking Time: 10 minutes
Optavia Counts: 1 lean/ 3 green/ 3 healthy fat/ 8 condiments
Ingredients:

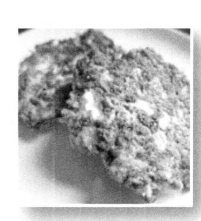

- 2 garlic cloves, minced
- ½ yellow onions, chopped
- 1/3 scallions, chopped
- 6 carrots, grated
- 1 tsp. cumin, ground
- ½ tsp. turmeric powder
- Salt and black pepper to the taste
- ¼ tsp. coriander, ground
- 1 tbsp. parsley, chopped
- ¼ tsp. lemon juice
- ½ cup almond flour
- 1 medium beets, peeled and grated
- 3 eggs, whisked
- ¼ cup tapioca flour
- 1 tbsp. olive oil

Directions:

1. In a bowl, combine the garlic with the onions, scallions, and the rest of the ingredients except the oil. Stir well and shape medium fritters out of this mix. Heat oil in a pan over medium-high fire. Add the fritters, cook for 5 minutes on each side, arrange on a platter and serve.

Nutrition: Calories: 209; Fat: 11.2 g; Fiber: 3 g; Carbs: 4.4 g; Protein: 4.8 g.

184. Asparagus with Garlic

Serving: 4
Difficulty: 3
Preparation Time: 15 minutes.
Cooking Time: 45 minutes.
Optavia Counts: 1 lean/ 0 green/ 1 healthy fat/ 2 condiments
Ingredients:

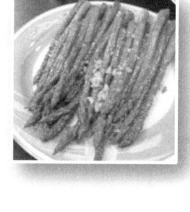

- 1 pound thick asparagus spears, trimmed and chopped
- ½ cup garlic cloves, peeled and chopped
- 3 tbsp. olive oil
- Salt and black pepper, to taste

Directions:

1. Mix asparagus with garlic, olive oil, black pepper and salt in a bowl. Cover and marinate for 30 minutes.
2. Meanwhile, at 450°F, preheat your oven. Spread the asparagus on a baking sheet.
3. Roast them for 15 minutes in the preheated oven.
4. Serve warm.
5. Suggestion: Serve the asparagus with toasted bread slices.

Variation Tip: Add boiled zucchini pasta to the mixture.
Nutrition Per Serving: Calories: 136; Fat: 10 g; Sodium: 249 mg; Carbs: 8 g; Fiber: 2 g; Sugar: 3 g; Protein: 4 g.

185. Black Beans and Sweet Potato Tacos

Serving: 4
Difficulty: 1
Preparation Time: 10 minutes
Cooking Time: 30 minutes
Optavia Counts: 1 lean/ 2 green/ 3 healthy fat/ 6 condiments
Ingredients:

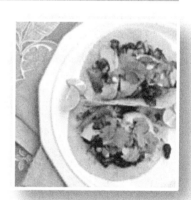

- 1-pound sweet potato (about 2 medium tsp.), remove skin and cut into ½-inch pieces
- 1 tbsp. olive oil, divided
- 1 tbsp. kosher salt, divided
- ¼ tsp. fresh black pepper on large white or yellow onion, finely chopped
- 1 tsp. red pepper
- 1 tsp. cumin
- 1 (15 oz.) can black beans, drained
- 1 cup water
- ¼ cup freshly chopped garlic
- 12 pieces Corn

To Serve:

- Guacamole
- Sliced cheese or feta cheese (optional)
- Wood Wedge

Directions:

1. In the oven, set out a tray in the middle rack and preheat to 425°F. Set a big sheet of aluminum foil on the work surface. Collect the tortillas from the top and wrap them completely in foil. Put it aside.
2. Put sweet potatoes on a small baking sheet. Mix with one tablespoon of oil and sprinkle with ½ teaspoon of salt and ¼ teaspoon of black pepper. Mix it properly and arrange it in a single layer on the sheet. Fry for 20 minutes. Cover the potatoes with a flat lid and set them aside.
3. Put the foil wrapping in the oven and continue cooking for about 10 minutes until the sweet potatoes are browned and stained and the seasonings are heated. Also, cook the beans.
4. Thereafter, heat one tablespoon of oil in a large skillet over low heat. Add the onions and cook, occasionally stirring, until translucent, about 3 minutes. Mix the pepper powder, cumin, and ½ teaspoon of salt. Add the beans and water.
5. Cover the pan and set the heat to low. Cook for 5 minutes, then slice and use the back of the fork to chop the beans a little, about half of the total. Continue cooking till the water content of the mixture is evaporated, and a semi-solid state is reached.
6. Peel the sweet potatoes and add the cantaloupe to the black beans and mix. Fill the taco cavity with a mixture of black beans and top with guacamole and cheese. Serve with lime wedges.

Nutrition: Calories: 251; Total fat: 4 g; Cholesterol: 94 mg; Fiber: 2 g; Protein: 15 g; Sodium: 329 mg.

186. Baked Portobello, Pasta, and Cheese

Serving: 4
Difficulty: 3
Preparation Time: 10 minutes
Cooking Time: 30 minutes
Optavia Counts: 1 lean/ 1 green/ 4 healthy fat/ 5 condiments
Ingredients:

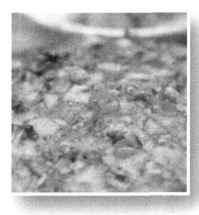

- 1 cup milk
- 1 cup vegan mozzarella cheese, shredded
- 1 large garlic clove, minced
- 1 tbsp. vegetable oil
- ¼ cup margarine
- ¼ tsp. basil, dried
- ¼- pound Portobello mushrooms, thinly sliced
- 1 tbsp. all-purpose flour - 1 tbsp. soy sauce
- 2 cups penne pasta, cooked according to manufacturer's directions for cooking
- 10 oz. frozen spinach, thawed, chopped

Directions:

1. Lightly, grease the baking pan of the Air Fryer with oil. For 2 minutes, heat to 360°F. Add mushrooms and cook for a minute. Transfer to a plate.
2. In the same pan, melt margarine for a minute. Stir in basil, garlic, and flour. Cook for 3 minutes. Stir and cook for another 2 minutes. Stir in half of the milk slowly while whisking continuously. Cook for another 2 minutes. Mix well. Cook for another 2 minutes. Stir in remaining milk and cook for another 3 minutes. Add cheese and mix well. Stir in soy sauce, spinach, mushrooms, and pasta. Mix well. Top with remaining cheese. Cook for 15 minutes at 390°F until tops are lightly browned.
3. Serve and enjoy.

Nutrition: Calories: 482; Carbs: 32.1 g; Protein: 16.0 g; Fat: 32.1 g.

CHAPTER 11.

PORK RECIPES

187. Pork Rind Nachos

Serving: 1
Difficulty: 1
Preparation Time: 5 minutes
Cooking Time: 5 minutes
Optavia Counts: 2 lean/ 1 green/ 2 healthy fat/ 0 condiments
Ingredients:

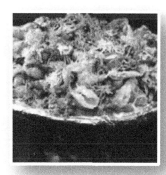

- 2 tbsp. of pork rinds (1 lean)
- ¼ cup shredded cooked chicken (½ lean)
- ½ cup shredded Monterey jack cheese (¼ healthy fat)
- ¼ cup sliced pickled jalapeños (¼ green)
- ¼ cup guacamole (¼ healthy fat)

Directions:

1. Place the pork rinds in a 6-inch round pan. Fill with grilled chicken and Monterey jack cheese. Place the pan in the basket with the Air Fryer. Set the temperature to 370°F and set the timer for 5 minutes or until the cheese has melted. Eat immediately with jalapeños, guacamole, and sour cream.

Nutrition: Calories: 295; Protein: 30 g; Fat: 27 g.

188. Air Fryer Whole Wheat Crusted Pork Chops

Serving: 1
Difficulty: 1
Preparation Time: 10 minutes
Cooking Time: 12 minutes
Optavia Counts: 2 lean/ 0 green/ 1 healthy fat/ 6 condiments
Ingredients:

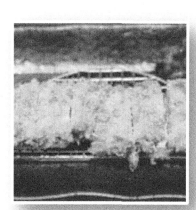

- 1 cup (½ healthy fat) whole-wheat breadcrumbs
- ¼ tsp. salt (¼ condiment)
- 2-4 pieces (center cut and boneless) pork chops (2 leans)
- ½ tsp. chili powder (¼ condiment)
- 1 tbsp. parmesan cheese (¼ healthy fat)
- 1 ½ tsp. paprika (½ condiment)
- 1 beaten egg (1 healthy fat)
- ½ tsp. onion powder (¼ condiment)
- ½ tsp. granulated garlic (¼ condiment)

Directions:

1. Allow the Air Fryer to preheat to 400°F. Rub kosher salt on each side of the pork chops, let them rest.
2. Add the beaten egg to a large bowl. Add the parmesan, breadcrumbs, garlic, pepper, paprika, chili powder and onion powder to a bowl and mix well. Put it in the Air Fryer and spray it with oil.
3. Leave to cook for 12 minutes at 400 F. Turn it upside down halfway through cooking. Cook for another six minutes. Serve with salad.

Nutrition: Calories: 425; Fat: 20 g; Protein: 31 g.

189. Pork Chop with Brussels Sprout

Serving: 1
Difficulty: 3
Preparation Time: 20 minutes
Cooking Time: 35 minutes
Optavia Counts: 1 lean/ 1 green/ 2 healthy fat/ 4 condiments
Ingredients:

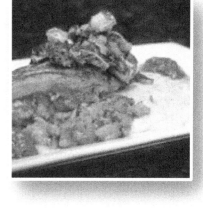

- 8 oz. pork chops
- 6 oz. Brussels sprouts
- Olive oil spray - 1 tsp. olive oil
- ⅛ tsp. kosher salt
- 1 tsp. maple syrup
- ½ tsp. black pepper
- 1 tsp. Dijon mustard

Directions:

1. Coat pork chop with olive oil cooking spray; sprinkle it with salt and ¼ teaspoon of the pepper. Mix together oil, syrup, mustard, and the remaining ¼ teaspoon of pepper in a bowl; add Brussels sprouts; coat it. Put pork chop on 1 side of the Air Fryer toaster oven tray and coated Brussels sprouts on the other side. Heat Air Fryer to 400°F, and cook until unless golden brown and pork is cooked to the required temperature.

Nutrition: Calories: 337; Fat: 11 g; Protein: 40 g; Carbs: 21 g.

190. Pork Dumplings with Sauce

Serving: 1
Difficulty: 4
Preparation Time: 20 minutes
Cooking Time: 60 minutes
Optavia Counts: 1 lean/ 3 green/ 3 healthy fat/ 6 condiments
Ingredients:

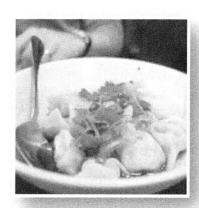

- 4 cups chopped Bok Choy
- 2 tsp. soy sauce
- 4 oz. ground pork
- 1 tsp. canola oil
- ¼ tsp. red pepper
- Olive oil spray
- 18 dumpling wrappers
- 1 tbsp. garlic - 1 tsp. Sesame oil
- ½ tsp. brown sugar - 1 tbsp. ginger
- 1 tbsp. chopped Scallions
- 2 tbsp. rice vinegar

Directions:

1. Put canola oil in a skillet over medium to high heat. Put bok choy, and cook, mixing often, until unless wilted and mostly dry, 6 to 8 minutes. Put ginger and garlic; cook, mixing constantly, 1 minute. Shift bok choy mixture to a plate to cool it for 5 minutes. Pat down the mixture dry with a paper towel. Fold the wrapper over to make a half-moon shape, pressing corners to seal. Do the same with the remaining wrappers and filling. Coat the Air Fryer toaster oven tray with olive oil spray. Put 6 dumplings in a tray, leaving room between each; spray the dumplings with olive oil spray.

Nutrition: Calories: 140; Fat: 5 g; Protein: 7 g; Carbs: 16 g.

191. Mozzarella Pork Belly Cheese

Serving: 1
Difficulty: 3
Preparation Time: 10 minutes
Cooking Time: 35 minutes
Optavia Counts: 1 lean/ 2 green/ 2 healthy fat/ 5 condiments
Ingredients:

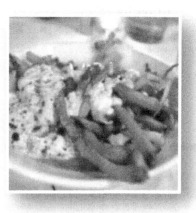

- 3 tsp. olive oil
- 8 basil leaves
- 8 oz. pork belly
- 2 tomatoes - ½ tsp. dried thyme
- ½ tsp. salt
- 1 tsp. dried oregano
- 1 tsp. dried basil - ½ tsp. black pepper
- 4 oz. mozzarella cheese

Directions:

1. Dry pork belly using paper towels and discard them. Brush olive oil over the pork belly. Put seasonings, and mix pork belly to coat all of it with seasonings. Now open pork belly, line 4 pieces, and top with about 4 slices of tomatoes and 4 basil leaves. Close down the pork belly and seal it with 4 toothpicks at the corners of the pork belly. Do the same with another pork belly. Spritz Air Fryer basket with olive oil cooking spray. Lay the pork belly. Coat the top of the pork belly with olive oil cooking spray for a golden color. Set down the temperature to 360°F and the set timer for 28 minutes or a bit more for desired crispness and a golden-brown color. When time completes, remove pork belly from baskets, and take out the toothpicks before serving. Garnish them with chopped basil.

Nutrition: Calories: 267; Fat: 20 g; Protein: 12 g; Carbs: 5 g; Fiber: 0.5 g.

192. Panko Crusted Pork Chops

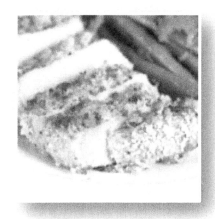

Serving: 2
Difficulty: 2
Preparation Time: 10 minutes
Cooking Time: 22 minutes
Optavia Counts: 2 lean/ 0 green/ 1 healthy fat/ 7 condiments
Ingredients:

- ¼ tsp. salt
- ¼ tsp. pepper
- 4 Boneless pork chops
- 1 egg beaten
- 1 tbsp. Parmesan cheese
- 1 cup panko
- ½ tsp. granulated garlic
- ½ tsp. paprika
- ½ tsp. onion powder
- ½ tsp. chili powder

Directions:

1. Preheat the Air Fryer toaster oven to 400°F while you prepare the pork chops. Spritz pork chops with salt on both sides and let it sit while you are preparing the seasonings and egg wash. Put the beaten egg in a bowl. Flip the pork chops over after 6 minutes if needed, coat with more olive oil spray and keep cooking for the remaining 6 minutes.

Nutrition: Calories: 220; Fat: 6 g; Protein: 27 g; Carbs: 13 g.

193. Apple Stuffy Pork Chop

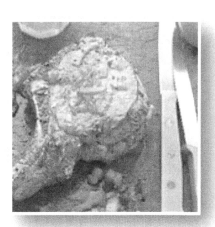

Serving: 2
Difficulty: 3
Preparation Time: 20 minutes
Cooking Time: 40 minutes
Servings: 4
Optavia Counts: 1 lean/ 0 green/ 1 healthy fat/ 15 condiments
Ingredients:

- 4 Boneless pork chops - 2 tsp. salt
- ½ tsp. dried sage
- ¼ tsp. nutmeg
- ½ tsp. garlic powder
- 1 apple sliced
- ¼ tsp. cinnamon
- ¼ tsp. paprika
- ¼ tsp. ground nutmeg
- ½ onion
- ¼ tsp. black pepper
- ½ tsp. dried sage
- 2 tsp. maple syrup
- ¼ tsp. cinnamon
- 2 tsp. Dijon mustard
- ½ tbsp. light butter
- ¼ cup celery chopped
- ½ tsp. garlic powder

Directions:

1. Pound the pork to ¾-inch thickness. In a bowl, mix Dijon mustard and maple syrup. Set it aside. Put remaining pork ingredients. Slice a deep pocket in pork chops, but be careful not to cut all the way through. Brush spice mixture all over and inside pork chops. In a skillet, melt the butter on medium to high heat. Put apples, onion, celery, and spiced for the apple stuffing. Mix it well. Cover it and cook for 8-10 minutes or until soft, stirring occasionally. Now fill each pocket with ¼ of the stuffing mixture.
2. Preheat Air Fryer toaster oven to 400°F. Coat basket with olive oil cooking spray. Put pork chops in a basket and air fry it for 3 minutes. Turn pork chops, brush with maple syrup/Dijon mixture, and air fry for about another 4 minutes if needed.

Nutrition: Calories: 378; Fat: 13 g; Protein: 33 g; Carbs: 8 g.

194. Air Fryer Pork Chop & Broccoli

Serving: 2
Difficulty: 2
Preparation Time: 20 minutes
Cooking Time: 20 minutes
Optavia Counts: 1 lean/ 1 green/ 1 healthy fat/ 5 condiments
Ingredients:

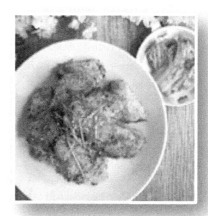

- 2 cups broccoli florets (1 green)
- 2 pieces bone-in pork chop (1 lean)
- ½ tsp. paprika (¼ condiment)
- 2 tbsp. avocado oil (1 healthy fat)
- ½ tsp. garlic powder (¼ condiment)
- ½ tsp. onion powder (¼ condiment)
- 2 cloves of crushed garlic (¼ condiment)
- 1 tsp. salt divided (¼ condiment)

Directions:

1. Let the Air Fryer preheat to 350°F. Spray the basket with cooking oil.
2. Add a tablespoon of oil, onion powder, half a teaspoon of salt, garlic powder and paprika in a bowl; mix well. Rub this spice mixture on the sides of the pork chop.
3. Add the pork chops to the fryer basket and cook for five minutes.
4. Turn the pork chop and add the broccoli; let it cook for another five minutes.
5. Remove from Air Fryer and serve.

Nutrition: Calories: 483; Fat: 20 g; Protein: 23 g.

195. Juicy Pork Chops

Serving: 2
Difficulty: 3
Preparation Time: 10 minutes
Cooking Time: 30 minutes
Optavia Counts: 1 lean/ 0 green/ 1 healthy fat/ 3 condiments
Ingredients:

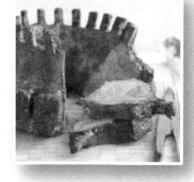

- 3 (6-oz.) pork chops
- 2 tsp. olive oil
- Salt & pepper
- Garlic powder
- Smoked paprika

Directions:

1. Coat lightly the pork chops with olive oil. Season them with salt, pepper, garlic powder, and smoked paprika. Put in the Air Fryer toaster oven and cook at 380°F for 10-14 minutes, turning the pork chops at the halfway cooking point if needed. Check it if cooked, and if not, then cook a little more if desired. Serve warm.

Nutrition: Calories: 287; Fat: 10 g; Protein: 35 g; Carbs: 6 g.

196. Super Easy Pork Chops

Serving: 3
Difficulty: 5
Preparation Time: 30 minutes
Cooking Time: 30 minutes
Optavia Counts: 1 lean/ 0 green/ 0 healthy fat/ 5 condiments
Ingredients:

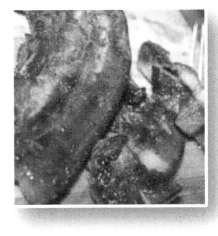

- 4 pork chops
- 2 tsp. salt
- 1 tsp. paprika
- 1 tsp. garlic powder
- 1 tsp. onion powder
- 1 tsp. oregano

Directions:

1. Preheat the oven to 350°F (175°C).
2. Clean and rinse the pork chops so the beef does not have extra water.
3. Combine herbs and spices using a Ziplock container.
4. Place one chop of pork in the zip lock bag at a time, seal, and shake until the chop of pork is thoroughly covered. Then put the pork chop on a wire rack over a parchment paper.
5. Repeat the process with any pork chop.
6. Place them in the oven and bake for 30 minutes.

Nutrition Per Serving: Calories: 200; Fat: 7 g; Net Carbs: 1 g; Protein: 34 g.

197. No Bread Pork Belly

Serving: 4
Difficulty: 4
Preparation Time: 15 minutes
Cooking Time: 95 minutes
Optavia Counts: 1 lean/ 0 green/ 1 healthy fat/ 6 condiments
Ingredients:

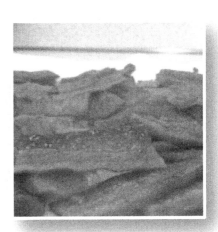

- Kosher salt
- Olive oil spray
- 12 oz. pork belly
- ½ tsp. parsley
- ¾ tsp. garlic powder
- ⅛ cayenne pepper
- ¾ tsp. onion powder
- ½ tsp. paprika

Directions:

1. Slice the pork belly to even pieces.
2. Fill a bowl with 6 cups of light warm water and include ¼ cup kosher salt, mix to dissolve.
3. Put the pork belly in the water and let them sit, refrigerate it for at least 1 to 1 ½ hours to brine. Take it out from the water, pat dry with paper towels, and remove the water.
4. In a bowl, add ¾ teaspoon of salt, with the left spices. Spray the pork with oil and rub it all over, then rub the spice mix over the pork. Preheat the Air Fryer toaster oven to 350°F.
5. Now heat an oven-safe or cast-iron skillet over high flame for 5 minutes until it becomes hot. Put the pork on the hot skillet, and cook it for 1 more minute. Rotate, and cook 1 minute from the other side. Shift the skillet to the oven and bake it until unless no longer pink in the center and the juices run clear, and a thermometer reads 165°F inserted in the center, about 8 to 10 minutes. You can cook it a little bit more for the desired crispness.

Nutrition: Calories: 258; Fat: 14 g; Protein: 29 g; Carbs: 5 g.

198. Creamy Pork Belly Rolls

Serving: 3
Difficulty: 4
Preparation Time: 20 minutes
Cooking Time: 55 minutes
Optavia Counts: 2 lean/ 2 green/ 3 healthy fat/ 1 condiments
Ingredients:

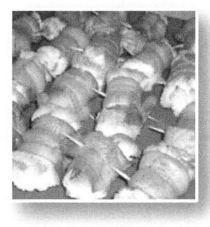

- 16 oz. pork belly
- Olive oil spray
- 2 oz. cream cheese
- ½ cup hot sauce
- ⅓ cup shredded carrots
- ½ cup blue cheese
- ⅓ cup chopped Scallions
- 16 egg roll wrappers

Directions:

1. Add pork belly to the slow cooker and put enough water or pork broth to cover it well. Cook it high for 4 hours. Take it out and shred it with two forks, remove the liquid. To prepare in the Instant Pot, put at least 1 cup broth or water, enough to cover the pork well.
2. Cook it on high pressure for 15 minutes on natural release. Remove liquid and shred it with two forks. During the time, add the cream cheese and hot sauce together until it is smooth. Put the pork, blue cheese, carrots and scallions and stir well, makes 3 cups. Place egg roll wrapper at a time on a clean surface, points facing top and bottom like a diamond. Spread 3 tablespoons of the buffalo dip mixture onto the bottom third of the wrapper.
3. Dip down your finger in a bowl of water and rub it along the edges of the wrapper. Lift the nearest point to you and wrap it around the filling. Wrap the left and right corners toward the center and continue to roll into an air-tight cylinder. Leave aside and do the same with the remaining wrappers and filling. Grease all sides of the egg rolls with olive oil spray using your fingers to equally coat.
4. Preheat the Air Fryer toaster oven to 400F. Spritz a sheet pan with oil. Shift the egg rolls to the baking sheet and cook until unless browned and crisp, about 16 to 18 minutes, flipping halfway if needed. Eat immediately, with dipping sauce on the side, if needed. You can cook it more for the desired crispness.

Nutrition: Calories: 305; Fat: 16 g; Protein: 16 g; Carbs: 24 g.

199. Seasoned Bleu Pork Belly

Serving: 3
Difficulty: 2
Preparation Time: 15 minutes
Cooking Time: 35 minutes
Optavia Counts: 3 lean/ 2 green/ 1 healthy fat/ 3 condiments
Ingredients:

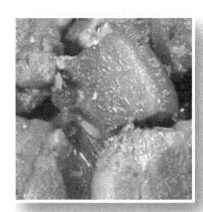

- 36 oz. pork belly
- ½ cup seasoned breadcrumb
- 2 large egg whites
- 1 large egg
- Salt and pepper
- Cooking spray
- 4.4 oz. cheese

Directions:

1. Preheat Air Fryer toaster oven to 450°F. Grease a large baking sheet with cooking spray. Wash down and dry the pork cutlets; lightly pound the pork to make thinner and lightly season with salt and pepper. Put pork onto the baking sheet seems side down. Spray the top of the pork with more olive oil spray and bake it for about 25 minutes, or until your desired crispness and golden brownish color.

Nutrition: Calories: 356; Fat: 20 g; Protein: 27 g; Carbs: 8 g.

200. Mustard Glazed Air Fryer Pork Tenderloin

Serving: 3
Difficulty: 1
Preparation Time: 10 minutes
Cooking Time: 18 minutes
Optavia Counts: 1 lean/ 0 green/ 0 healthy fat/ 7 condiments
Ingredients:

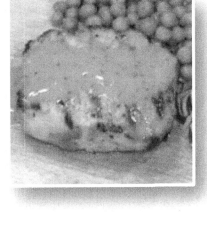

- ¼ cup yellow mustard (½ green)
- 1 pork tenderloin (1 lean)
- ¼ tsp salt (¼ condiment)
- 3 tbsp. honey (½ healthy fat)
- ⅛ tsp. black pepper (¼ condiment)
- 1 tbsp. minced garlic (¼ condiment)
- 1 tsp. dried rosemary (¼ green)
- 1 tsp. Italian seasoning (⅛ condiment)

Directions:
1. Using a knife, cut the top of the pork tenderloin. Add the garlic (minced) into the cuts. Then sprinkle with kosher salt and pepper.
2. In a bowl, add the honey, mustard, rosemary, and Italian seasoning mixture until well blended. Rub this mustard mix all over the pork.
3. Place the pork tenderloin in the basket of the Air Fryer. Cook for 18-20 minutes at 400°F. With an instant-read thermometer, verify that the internal temperature of the pig should be 145°F.
4. Remove from Air Fryer and serve with a side of salad.

Nutrition: Calories: 390; Protein: 59 g; Fat: 11 g.

201. Rustic Pork Ribs

Serving: 3
Difficulty: 2
Preparation Time: 5 minutes
Cooking Time: 25 minutes
Optavia Counts: 1 lean/ 0 green/ 1 healthy fat/ 8 condiments
Ingredients:

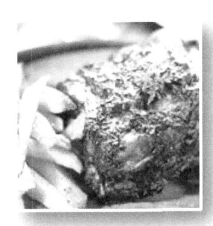

- 1 rack of pork ribs
- 3 tbsp. dry red wine
- 1 tbsp. soy sauce
- ½ tsp. dried thyme
- ½ tsp. onion powder
- ½ tsp. garlic powder
- ½ tsp. ground black pepper
- 1 tsp. smoke salt
- 1 tbsp. cornstarch
- ½ tsp. olive oil

Directions:
1. Begin by preheating your Air Fryer oven to 390°F. Place all ingredients in a mixing bowl and let them marinate for at least 1 hour.
2. Put it into the oven rack/basket. Place the rack on the middle-shelf of the Air Fryer oven. Set temperature to 390°F, and time to 25 minutes. Cook the marinated ribs for approximately 25 minutes.
3. Serve hot.

Nutrition: Calories: 268; Fat: 16 g; Protein: 24 g; Carbs: 7 g.

202. Pork Tenderloin

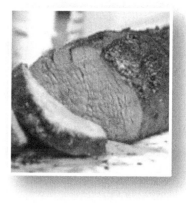

Serving: 3
Difficulty: 3
Preparation Time: 10 minutes
Cooking Time: 25 minutes
Optavia Counts: 1 lean/ 0 green/ 1 healthy fat/ 2 condiments
Ingredients:

- 1 ½ pounds pork tenderloin
- 1 tbsp. olive oil
- ¼ tsp. garlic powder
- ¼ tsp. salt

Directions:

1. Brine the tenderloin according to brining instructions (this is optional). Take tenderloin out from the fridge 20 minutes before cooking. If it was brined, discard brine and rinse pork. Cut silver skin according to these given instructions.
2. Preheat Air Fryer toaster oven to 450F. In a bowl, mix olive oil, black pepper, and garlic powder. Add the salt If you did not brine the pork. Stir. Brush olive oil mixture all over tenderloin. Put tenderloin in the Air Fryer tray, bending it if needed for it to fit. Cook it for 10 minutes, or until it has reached the desired doneness as indicated on an instant-read thermometer, 145-160F has been recommended by the US Pork Board. This will take 8 to 15 extra minutes. Set aside for at least 5 minutes before slicing into ½-to-¾-inch pieces. Serve immediately.

Nutrition: Calories: 321; Fat: 28 g; Carbs: 7 g; Protein: 42 g.

203. Quick Pork Belly

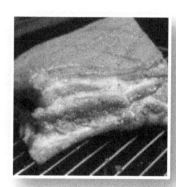

Serving: 4
Difficulty: 4
Preparation Time: 20 minutes
Cooking Time: 65 minutes
Optavia Counts: 1 lean/ 0 green/ 1 healthy fat/ 1 condiments
Ingredients:

- 2 pounds piece of pork belly
- Olive oil spray
- Salt

Directions:

1. Take out the pork belly; if you are using a packaged piece of pork belly, then there is no need to dry the skin.
2. Score the skin with a sharp knife by slicing the rind and taking care not to cut through to the meat underneath.
3. Put on the tray inside your Air Fryer toaster oven, rind side up. Coat evenly with olive oil cooking spray.
4. Cover it evenly and thickly with a layer of cracked salt. Set your Air Fryer toaster oven to 180°C/356 F for 45 minutes. Then check the pork belly, if you see one side cooking faster than the other, it can be a good idea to flip the rack 180 degrees.
5. Now turn the Air Fryer up to full (230°C/446F) and set more 15 minutes. Some pieces of pork will be ready after these steps, others might need more than 15 minutes. Your pork belly will be done when the crackling is hard and crispy.
6. Different Air Fryers can have their own cooking times, so be aware of this when making your pork belly. Some Air Fryers toaster oven may require more or less cooking time.

Nutrition: Calories: 390; Fat: 20 g; Carbs: 3 g; Protein: 34 g.

204. Crispy Pork Cutlets

Serving: 4
Difficulty: 4
Preparation Time: 10 minutes
Cooking Time: 20 minutes
Optavia Counts: 2 lean/ 0 green/ 0 healthy fat/ 7 condiments
Ingredients:

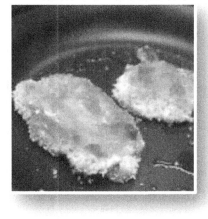

- 1 pound boneless pork chops
- ¼ cup flour
- ¼ tsp. pepper
- ½ tsp. salt
- ¾ cup panko breadcrumbs
- 2 eggs
- 2 tbsp. mayonnaise
- 2 tsp. Dijon
- ½ tsp. apple cider vinegar
- 2 tsp. honey

Directions:

1. Between the two layers of saran wrap; equally, pound the pork chops until unless they are ¼ inch thick. Put the flour, salt, and pepper to a plate and mix with a fork until well mixed. In a bowl, whisk the two eggs. On another plate, add the Panko breadcrumbs. Dip down each pork cutlet into the flour, shaking off any extra. Then dip down the floured pork into the egg wash. Now, dip the pork into the breadcrumbs. Press the meat into the breadcrumbs so there can be a good coating. Arrange the cutlets in the Air Fryer toaster oven and cook it at 390°F for 10 to 12 minutes, or until unless the pork reaches an internal temperature of 165°F. During cooking, prepare the honey Dijon dipping sauce, but mixing all of the ingredients together. Eat the cooked pork with the sauce.

Nutrition: Calories: 190; Carbs: 33 g; Fat: 4 g; Protein: 6 g.

205. Southern Style Pork Chops

Serving: 4
Difficulty: 2
Preparation Time: 10 minutes
Cooking Time: 25 minutes
Optavia Counts: 1 lean/ 0 green/ 1 healthy fat/ 5 condiments
Ingredients:

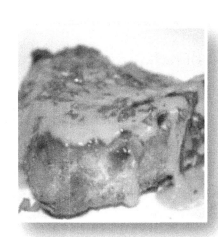

- 3 tbsp. buttermilk
- 4 pork chops
- Seasoning salt to taste
- ¼ cup flour
- Pork seasoning
- 1 Ziploc bag
- Cooking oil spray
- Pepper to taste

Directions:

1. Wash the pork chops and pat dry them. With the seasoning salt and pepper, season the pork chops. Pour the buttermilk over the pork chops. Put the pork chops in a Ziploc baggie with flour. Shake it to coat it completely. Marinate it for 30 minutes. Put the pork chops in the Air Fryer toaster oven. Spray the pork chops with cooking oil spray. Cook the pork chops at 380°F for 15 minutes. Turn the pork chops over to the other side after 10 minutes.

Nutrition: Calories: 173; Fat: 6 g; Protein: 22 g; Carbs: 7 g.

206. Roasted Pepper Pork Prosciutto

Serving: 4
Difficulty: 3
Preparation Time: 20 minutes
Cooking Time: 60 minutes
Optavia Counts: 2 lean/ 2 green/ 3 healthy fat/ 3 condiments
Ingredients:

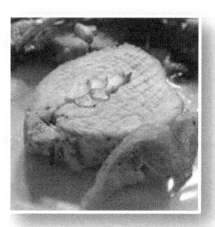

- 24 oz. pork cutlets
- Olive oil spray
- 12 oz. slices thin prosciutto
- 4 slices mozzarella
- 22 oz. roasted peppers
- 1 lemon
- 24 Spinach leaves
- 1 tbsp. olive oil
- ½ cup GF breadcrumbs
- Salt and fresh pepper

Directions:

1. First, wash and dry the pork cutlets very well with paper towels. Add breadcrumbs to a bowl and in another second bowl, stir the olive oil, lemon juice, and pepper. Preheat the Air Fryer toaster oven to 450°F. Slightly coat a baking dish with olive oil spray.
2. Put each cutlet on a work surface such as a cutting board and lay ½ slice prosciutto, ½ slice cheese, 1 piece of roasted pepper, and 3 spinach leaves on one side of the pork cutlet. Roll it and put the seam side down on a dish.
3. Dip down the pork in the olive oil and lemon juice; after that, into the breadcrumbs. Do the same with the pork left. Bake it for 25 to 30 minutes or until your desired crispness.

Nutrition: Calories: 268; Fat: 16 g; Protein: 24 g; Carbs: 7 g; Fiber: 1 g.

207. Easy Cook Pork

Serving: 4
Difficulty: 3
Preparation Time: 15 minutes
Cooking Time: 45 minutes
Optavia Counts: 1 lean/ 0 green/ 1 healthy fat/ 4 condiments
Ingredients:

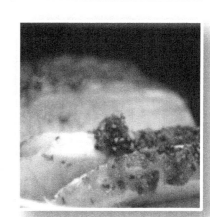

- ¼ tsp. garlic powder
- ½ tsp. salt
- ¼ tsp. smoked paprika
- 2 tbsp. butter
- ¼ tsp. black pepper
- 4 boneless skinless Pork

Directions:

1. In a bowl, mix butter, salt, garlic powder, smoked paprika, and pepper. Rub both sides of pork with butter mixture.
2. Put the pork in an Air Fryer toaster oven tray, standing against the sides of the basket if needed. Set it to 350°F; cook it for 15 minutes or until the juice of pork is clear when the center of the thickest part is cut (at least 165°F). You can cook it a little bit more for the desired crispness.

Nutrition: Calories: 362; Fat: 21 g; Protein: 30 g; Carbs: 4 g.

CHAPTER 12.

APPETIZER RECIPES

208. Cauliflower Rice

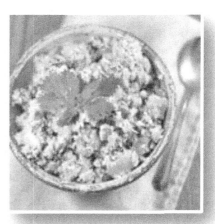

Serving: 1
Difficulty: 3
Preparation Time: 5 minutes
Cooking Time: 20 minutes
Optavia Counts: 0 lean/ 5 green/ 2 healthy fat/ 4 condiments
Ingredients:
Round 1:

- ½ tsp. turmeric
- ½ cup diced carrot
- ½ tbsp. low-sodium soy sauce
- ⅛ block extra firm tofu

Round 2:

- ¼ minced garlic cloves
- ½ cup chopped broccoli
- ½ tbsp. minced ginger
- ¼ tbsp. rice vinegar
- ¼ tsp. toasted sesame oil
- ½ tbsp. reduced-sodium soy sauce
- ½ cup rice cauliflower

Directions:

1. Crush tofu in a large bowl and toss with all the Round 1 ingredients.
2. Lock the Air Fryer lid—Preheat the Instant Crisp Air Fryer to 370°F. Also, set the temperature to 370°F, set the time to 10 minutes, and cook 10 minutes, making sure to shake once.
3. In another bowl, toss ingredients from Round 2 together.
4. Add Round 2 mixture to Instant Crisp Air Fryer and cook another 10 minutes to shake 5 minutes.

Nutrition: Calories: 67; Fat: 8 g; Protein: 3 g.

209. Bell-Pepper Wrapped in Tortilla

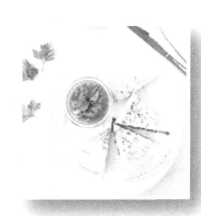

Serving: 1
Difficulty: 1
Preparation Time: 5 minutes
Cooking Time: 15 minutes
Optavia Counts: 1 lean/ 2 green/ 1 healthy fat/ 1 condiments
Ingredients:

- ¼ small red bell pepper
- ¼ tbsp. water
- 1 large tortilla
- 1-piece commercial vegan nuggets, chopped
- Mixed greens for garnish

Directions:

1. Preheat the Instant Crisp Air Fryer to 400°F.
2. In a skillet heated over medium flame, water sauté the vegan nuggets and bell peppers. Set aside.
3. Place filling inside the corn tortillas.
4. Fold the tortillas, place them inside the Instant Crisp Air Fryer, and cook for 15 minutes until the tortilla wraps are crispy.
5. Serve with mixed greens on top.

Nutrition: Calories: 548; Fat: 21 g; Protein: 46 g.

210. Zucchini Omelet

Serving: 1
Difficulty: 1
Preparation Time: 10 minutes
Cooking Time: 10 minutes
Servings: 1
Optavia Counts: 1 lean/ 3 green/ 1 healthy fat/ 1 condiments
Ingredients:

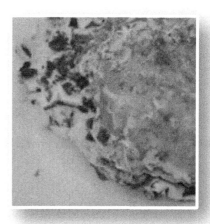

- ½ tsp. butter (1 healthy fat)
- ½ zucchini, julienned (1 green)
- 1 egg (1 lean)
- ⅛ tsp. fresh basil, chopped (¼ green)
- ⅛ tsp. red pepper flakes (¼ green)
- Salted and newly ground black pepper to taste (½ condiment)

Directions:

1. Preheat the Instant Crisp Air Fryer to 355°F.
2. Melt butter on a medium heat using a skillet.
3. Add zucchini and cook for about 3-4 minutes.
4. In a bowl, add the eggs, basil, red pepper flakes, salt, and black pepper and beat well.
5. Add cooked zucchini and gently stir to combine.
6. Transfer the mixture into the Instant Crisp Air Fryer pan. Lock the Air Fryer lid.
7. Cook for about 10 minutes. Also, you may opt to wait until it is done thoroughly.

Nutrition: Calories: 281; Fat: 21 g; Protein: 9 g.

211. Cheesy Cauliflower Fritters

Serving: 1
Difficulty: 3
Preparation Time: 10 minutes
Cooking Time: 7 minutes
Optavia Counts: 0 lean/ 4 green/ 4 healthy fat/ 0 condiments
Ingredients:

- ½ cup chopped parsley
- 1 cup Italian breadcrumbs
- ⅓ cup shredded mozzarella cheese
- ⅓ cup shredded sharp cheddar cheese
- 1 egg
- 3 minced garlic cloves
- 2 tbsp. chopped scallions
- 1 head of cauliflower

Directions:

1. Preparing the Ingredients. Cut the cauliflower up into florets. Wash well and pat dry. Place into a food processor and pulse 20-30 seconds till it looks like rice.
2. Place the cauliflower rice in a bowl and mix with pepper, salt, egg, cheeses, breadcrumbs, garlic, and scallions.
3. With hands, form 15 patties of the mixture and then add more breadcrumbs if needed.
4. With olive oil, spritz patties, and put the fitters into your Instant Crisp Air Fryer. Pile it into a single layer. Lock the Air Fryer lid. Set temperature to 390°F, and time to 7 minutes, flipping after 7 minutes.

Nutrition: Calories: 209; Fat: 17 g; Protein: 6 g.

212. Zucchini Parmesan Chips

Serving: 1
Difficulty: 1
Preparation Time: 10 minutes
Cooking Time: 8 minutes
Optavia Counts: 0 lean/ 1 green/ 3 healthy fat/ 1 condiments
Ingredients:

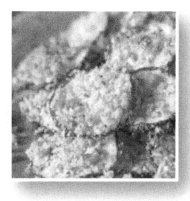

- ½ tsp. paprika
- ½ cup grated parmesan cheese
- ½ cup Italian breadcrumbs
- Lightly beaten egg
- Thinly sliced zucchinis

Directions:

1. Use a very sharp knife or mandolin slicer to slice zucchini as thinly as you can. Pat off extra moisture.
2. Beat egg with a pinch of pepper and salt and a bit of water.
3. Combine paprika, cheese, and breadcrumbs in a bowl.
4. Dip slices of zucchini into the egg mixture and then into the breadcrumb mixture. Press gently to coat.
5. Mist with olive oil cooking spray encrusted zucchini slices. Put into your Instant Crisp Air Fryer in a single layer. Latch the Air Fryer lid. Set temperature to 350°F and set time to 8 minutes.
6. Sprinkle with salt and serve with salsa.

Nutrition: Calories: 211; Fat: 16 g; Protein: 8 g.

213. Jalapeno Cheese Balls

Serving: 1
Difficulty: 1
Preparation Time: 10 minutes
Cooking Time: 8 minutes
Optavia Counts: 0 lean/ 1 green/ 5 healthy fat/ 1 condiments
Ingredients:

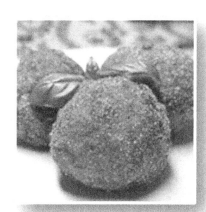

- 8 oz. cream cheese (2 healthy fats)
- 1/6 cup shredded mozzarella cheese (⅓ healthy fat)
- 1/6 cup shredded Cheddar cheese (⅓ healthy fat)
- ½ Jalapeños, finely chopped (1 green)
- ½ cup breadcrumbs (1 healthy fat)
- 2 eggs (4 healthy fats)
- ½ cup all-purpose flour (1 healthy fat)
- Salt (½ condiment)
- Pepper (½ condiment)

Directions:

1. Combine the cream cheese, mozzarella, Cheddar, and jalapeños in a medium bowl. Mix well.
2. Form the cheese mixture into balls about an inch thick. You may also use a small ice cream scoop. It works well.
3. Arrange the cheese balls on a sheet pan and place them in the freezer for 15 minutes. It will help the cheese balls maintain their shape while frying.
4. Spray the Instant Crisp Air Fryer basket with cooking oil. Place the breadcrumbs in a small bowl. In another small bowl, beat the eggs. In the third small bowl, combine the flour with salt and pepper to taste, and mix well. Remove the cheese balls from the freezer. Plunge the cheese balls in the flour, then the eggs, and then the breadcrumbs.
5. Place the cheese balls in the Instant Crisp Air Fryer. Spray with cooking oil. Lock the Air Fryer lid and cook for 8 minutes.
6. Open the Instant Crisp Air Fryer and flip the cheese balls. I recommend flipping them instead of shaking, so the balls maintain their form. Cook an additional 4 minutes. Cool before serving.

Nutrition: Calories: 96; Fat: 6 g; Protein: 4 g.

214. Crispy Roasted Broccoli

Serving: 2
Difficulty: 1
Preparation Time: 10 minutes
Cooking Time: 8 minutes
Optavia Counts: 0 lean/ 1 green/ 2 healthy fat/ 4 condiments
Ingredients:

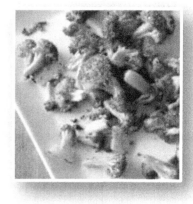

- ¼ tsp. masala (½ condiment)
- ½ tsp. red chili powder (1 condiment)
- ½ tsp. salt (1 condiment)
- ¼ tsp. turmeric powder (½ condiment)
- 1 tbsp. chickpea flour (1 healthy fat)
- 1 tbsp. yogurt (2 healthy fats)
- ½ Pound broccoli (1 green)

Directions:

1. Cut broccoli up into florets. Immerse in a bowl of water with 2 teaspoons of salt for at least half an hour to remove impurities.
2. Take out broccoli florets from water and let drain. Wipe down thoroughly.
3. Mix all other ingredients to create a marinade.
4. Toss broccoli florets in the marinade. Cover and chill for 15-30 minutes.
5. Preheat the Instant Crisp Air Fryer to 390°F. Place marinated broccoli florets into the fryer, lock the Air Fryer lid, set the temperature to 350°F, and the time to 10 minutes. Florets will be crispy when done.

Nutrition: Calories: 96; Fat: 1.3 g; Protein: 7 g.

215. Coconut Battered Cauliflower Bites

Serving: 2
Difficulty: 2
Preparation Time: 5 minutes
Cooking Time: 20 minutes
Optavia Counts: 1 lean/ 2 green/ 4 healthy fat/ 4 condiments
Ingredients:

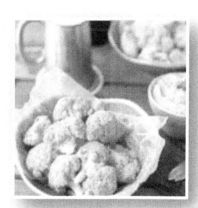

- Salt and pepper to taste
- Flax egg or 1 tbsp. flaxseed meal + 3 tbsp. water
- 1 small cauliflower, cut into florets
- 1 tsp. mixed spice
- ½ tsp. mustard powder
- 1 tbsp. maple syrup
- 1 clove of garlic, minced
- 1 tbsp. soy sauce
- ⅓ cup oats flour
- ⅓ cup plain flour
- ⅓ cup desiccated coconut

Directions:

1. In a mixing bowl, mix oats, flour, and desiccated coconut. Season with salt and pepper to taste. Set aside.
2. In another bowl, place the flax egg and add a pinch of salt to taste. Set aside.
3. Season the cauliflower with mixed spice and mustard powder.
4. Dredge the florets in the flax egg first, then in the flour mixture.
5. Place inside the Instant Crisp Air Fryer, lock the Air Fryer lid, and cook at 400°F or 15 minutes.
6. Meanwhile, place the maple syrup, garlic, and soy sauce in a saucepan and heat over medium flame. Wait for it to boil and adjust the heat to low until the sauce thickens.
7. After 15 minutes, take out the Instant Crisp Air Fryer's florets and place them in the saucepan.
8. Toss to coat the florets and place inside the Instant Crisp Air Fryer. Cook for another 5 minutes.

Nutrition: Calories: 154; Fat: 2.3 g; Protein: 4.6 g.

216. Crispy Jalapeno Coins

Serving: 2
Difficulty: 1
Preparation Time: 10 minutes
Cooking Time: 5 minutes
Optavia Counts: 0 lean/ 1 green/ 2 healthy fat/ 3 condiments

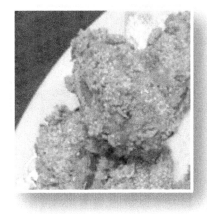

Ingredients:

- 1 egg
- 2-3 tbsp. coconut flour
- 1 sliced and seeded jalapeno
- Pinch of garlic powder
- Bit of Cajun seasoning (optional)
- Pinch of pepper and salt

Directions:

1. Preparing the Ingredients. Ensure your Instant Crisp Air Fryer is preheated to 400F.
2. Mix all dry ingredients.
3. Pat jalapeno slices dry. Dip coins into the egg wash and then into the dry mixture. Toss to coat thoroughly.
4. Add coated jalapeno slices to Instant Crisp Air Fryer in a singular layer. Spray with olive oil.
5. Lock the Air Fryer lid. Set temperature to 350°F and set time to 5 minutes. Cook just till crispy.

Nutrition: Calories: 128; Fat: 8 g; Protein: 7 g.

217. Buffalo Cauliflower

Serving: 2
Difficulty: 5
Preparation Time: 5 minutes
Cooking Time: 15 minutes
Optavia Counts: 0 lean/ 1 green/ 2 healthy fat/ 2 condiments

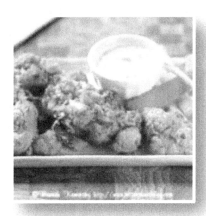

Ingredients:
Cauliflower:

- 1 cup panko breadcrumbs (1 healthy fat)
- 1 tsp. salt (1 condiment)
- 1 large head cauliflower florets (2 greens)

Buffalo Coating:

- ¼ cup Vegan Buffalo sauce (½ condiment)
- ¼ cup melted vegan butter (½ healthy fat)

Directions:

1. Melt butter in the microwave and whisk in buffalo sauce.
2. Dip each cauliflower floret into the buffalo mixture, ensuring it gets coated well. Holdover a bowl till the floret is done dripping.
3. Mix breadcrumbs with salt.
4. Dredge dipped florets into breadcrumbs and place them into Instant Crisp Air Fryer. Lock the Air Fryer lid. Set temperature to 350°F and time to 15 minutes. When slightly browned, they are ready to eat!
5. Serve with your favorite Keto dipping sauce!

Nutrition: Calories: 194; Fat: 17 g; Protein: 10 g.

218. Carrot Cake Oatmeal

Serving: 2
Difficulty: 2
Preparation Time: 10 minutes
Cooking Time: 15 minutes
Optavia Counts: 0 lean/ 1 green/ 5 healthy fat/ 3 condiments
Ingredients:

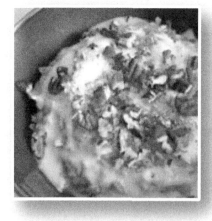

- ⅛ cup pecans (¼ healthy fat)
- ½ cup finely shredded carrot (1 green)
- ¼ cup old-fashioned oats (½ healthy fat)
- 5/8 cups unsweetened nondairy milk (¼ healthy fat)
- ½ tbsp. pure maple syrup (1 healthy fat)
- ½ tsp. ground cinnamon (1 condiment)
- ½ tsp. ground ginger (1 condiment)
- ⅛ tsp. ground nutmeg (¼ condiment)
- 1 tbsp. chia seed (1 healthy fat)

Directions:

1. Over medium-high heat in a skillet, toast the pecans for 3 to 4 minutes, often stirring, until browned and fragrant (watch closely, as they can burn quickly). Pour the pecans onto a cutting board and coarsely chop them. Set aside. Using an 8-quart pot at medium-high heat, combine the carrot, oats, milk, maple syrup, cinnamon, ginger, and nutmeg. When it is already boiling, reduce the heat to medium-low. Cook, uncovered, for 10 minutes, stirring occasionally.
2. Stir in the chopped pecans and chia seeds. Serve immediately.

Nutrition: Calories: 307; Fat: 17 g; Protein: 7 g.

219. Spiced Sorghum and Berries

Serving: 2
Difficulty: 2
Preparation Time: 5 minutes
Cooking Time: 1 hour
Optavia Counts: 2 lean/ 0 green/ 5 healthy fat/ 3 condiments
Ingredients:

- ¼ cup whole-grain sorghum
- ¼ tsp. ground cinnamon
- ¼ tsp. Chinese five-spice powder
- ¾ cups water
- ¼ cup non-dairy milk, unsweetened
- ¼ tsp. vanilla extract
- ½ tbsp. pure maple syrup
- ½ tbsp. chia seed
- ⅛ cup sliced almonds
- ½ cup fresh raspberries, divided

Directions:

1. Using a large pot over medium-high heat, stir together the sorghum, cinnamon, five-spice powder, and water. Wait for the water to a boil, cover the bank, and reduce the heat to medium-low. Cook for 1 hour, or until the sorghum is soft and chewy. If the sorghum grains are still hard, add another water cup and cook for 15 minutes more.
2. Using a glass measuring cup, whisk together the milk, vanilla, and maple syrup to blend. Add the mixture to the sorghum and the chia seeds, almonds, and 1 cup of raspberries. Gently stir to combine.
3. When serving, top with the remaining 1 cup of fresh raspberries.

Nutrition: Calories: 289; Fat: 8 g; Protein: 9 g.

220. Plant-Powered Pancakes

Serving: 3
Difficulty: 1
Preparation Time: 5 minutes
Cooking Time: 15 minutes
Optavia Counts: 0 lean/ 0 green/ 6 healthy fat/ 1 condiments
Ingredients:

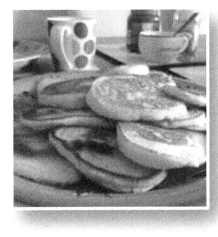

- 1 cup whole-wheat flour (1 healthy fat)
- 1 tsp. baking powder (½ healthy fat)
- ½ tsp. ground cinnamon (½ condiment)
- 1 cup plant-based milk (1 healthy fat)
- ½ cup unsweetened applesauce (1 healthy fat)
- ¼ cup maple syrup (½ healthy fat)
- 1 tsp. vanilla extract (1 healthy fat)

Directions:

1. In a large bowl, combine the flour, baking powder, and cinnamon.
2. Stir in the milk, applesauce, maple syrup, and vanilla until no dry flour is left, and the batter is smooth.
3. Preheat a huge, non-stick skillet over medium flame. For each pancake, pour ¼ cup of batter onto the hot skillet. Once bubbles form over the top of the pancake and the sides begin to brown, flip and cook for 1 to 2 minutes more. Repeat until all of the batters are used and serve.

Nutrition: Fat: 2 g; Protein: 5 g; Calories: 591.

221. Sweet Cashew Cheese Spread

Serving: 3
Difficulty: 1
Preparation Time: 5 minutes
Cooking Time: 5 minutes
Optavia Counts: 0 lean/ 0 green/ 1 healthy fat/ 2 condiments
Ingredients:

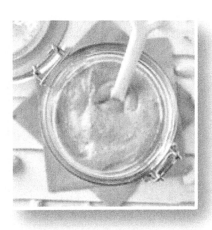

- 5 drops stevia (½ condiment)
- 2 cups cashews, raw (3 healthy fats)
- ½ cup water (1 condiment)

Directions:

1. Soak the cashews overnight in water.
2. Next, drain the excess water, then transfer cashews to a food processor.
3. Add in the stevia and the water.
4. Process until smooth.
5. Serve chilled. Enjoy.

Nutrition: Fat: 7 g; Protein: 7 g; Calories: 322.

222. Crispy Cauliflowers

Serving: 3
Difficulty: 1
Preparation Time: 10 minutes
Cooking Time: 10 minutes
Optavia Counts: 1 lean/ 3 green/ 2 healthy fat/ 5 condiments
Ingredients:

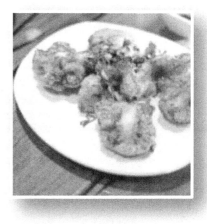

- 1 cup cauliflower florets, diced (6 greens)
- ½ cup almond flour (1 healthy fat)
- ½ cup coconut flour (1 healthy fat)
- Salt and pepper to taste (½ condiment)
- 1 tsp. mixed herbs (1 green)
- 1 tsp. chives, chopped (1 green)
- 1 egg (1 lean)
- 1 tsp. cumin (1 condiment)
- ½ tsp. garlic powder (1 condiment)
- 1 cup water (1 condiment)
- Oil for frying (1 condiment)

Directions:

1. Combine the egg, salt, garlic, water, cumin, chives, mixed herbs, pepper, and flour in a mixing bowl.
2. Stir in the cauliflower to the mixture and then fry them in oil until they become golden in color.
3. Serve.

Nutrition: Protein: 3.3 g; Fat: 10.4 g; Calories: 259.

223. Pesto Zucchini Noodles

Serving: 3
Difficulty: 3
Preparation Time: 10 minutes
Cooking Time: 30 minutes
Optavia Counts: 0 lean/ 2 green/ 2 healthy fat/ 5 condiments
Ingredients:

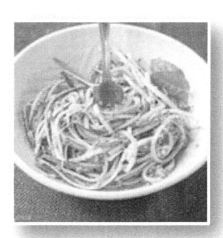

- 4 small zucchinis, spiralized
- 1 tbsp avocado oil
- 2 garlic cloves, chopped
- ⅔ cup olive oil
- ⅓ cup parmesan cheese, grated
- 2 cups fresh basil
- ⅓ cup almonds
- ⅛ tsp. black pepper
- ¾ tsp. sea salt

Directions:

1. Add zucchini noodles into a colander and sprinkle with ¼ teaspoon of salt.
2. Cover and let sit for 30 minutes.
3. Drain zucchini noodles well and pat dry.
4. Preheat the oven to 400°F.
5. Place almonds on a parchment-lined baking sheet and bake for 6-8 minutes.
6. Transfer toasted almonds into the food processor and process until coarse.
7. Add olive oil, cheese, basil, garlic, pepper, and remaining salt in a food processor with almonds and process until pesto texture.
8. Cook avocado oil in a large pan over medium-high heat.
9. Add zucchini noodles and cook for 4-5 minutes.
10. Pour pesto over zucchini noodles, mix well, and cook for 1 minute.
11. Serve immediately with baked salmon.

Nutrition: Calories: 525; Fat: 47 g; Protein: 17 g.

224. Herbed Wild Rice

Serving: 3
Difficulty: 5
Preparation Time: 10 minutes
Cooking Time: 4 to 6 hours
Optavia Counts: 1 lean/ 3 green/ 0 healthy fat/ 3 condiments
Ingredients:

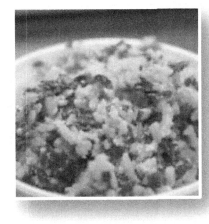

- 2 cups wild rice, rinsed and drained (2 lean)
- 2 cups Roasted Vegetable Broth (2 condiments)
- ½ tsp. salt (⅛ condiment)
- ½ tsp. dried thyme leaves (⅛ condiment)
- ½ tsp. dried basil leaves (¼ green)
- 2 bay leaf (¼ green)
- ⅓ cup fresh flat-leaf parsley (¼ green)

Directions:

1. In a 6-quart slow cooker, mix the wild rice, vegetable broth, salt, thyme, basil, and bay leaf.
2. Close and cook over low heat for 4 to 6 hours. You can cook this dish longer until the wild rice pops, taking about 7 to 8 hours. Remove and discard the bay leaf.
3. Stir in the parsley and serve.

Nutrition: Calories: 258; Fat: 2 g; Protein: 6 g.

225. Beef with Broccoli or Cauliflower Rice

Serving: 4
Difficulty: 2
Preparation Time: 10 minutes
Cooking Time: 30 minutes
Optavia Counts: 1 lean/ 2 green/ 0 healthy fat/ 4 condiments
Ingredients:

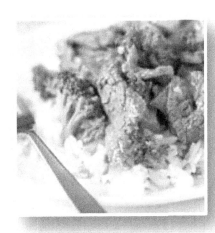

- 1 pound raw beef round steak, cut into strips (1 lean)
- 1 tbsp. + 2 tsp. low sodium soy sauce (¼ condiment)
- 1 Splenda packet (¼ condiment)
- ½ cup water (¼ condiment)
- 1 ½ cups broccoli florets (1 green)
- 1 tsp. sesame or olive oil (¼ condiment)
- 4 cups cooked, grated cauliflower or frozen riced cauliflower (1 green)

Directions:

1. Stir steak with soy sauce and let sit for about 15 minutes.
2. Heat oil over medium-high fire and stir-fry beef for 3-5 minutes or until browned.
3. Remove from pan. Place broccoli, Splenda, and water.
4. Cover and cook for 5 minutes or until broccoli starts to turn tender, stirring sometimes.
5. Add beef back in and heat up thoroughly.
6. Serve the dish with cauliflower rice.

Nutrition: Fats: 16 g; Protein: 9 g; Calories: 211.

226. Barley Risotto

Serving: 4
Difficulty: 2
Preparation Time: 15 minutes
Cooking Time: 7 to 8 hours
Optavia Counts: 0 lean/ 2 green/ 2 healthy fat/ 3 condiments
Ingredients:

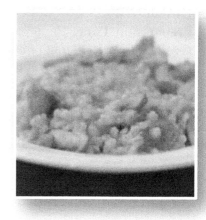

- ¼ cups hulled barley, rinsed (2 green)
- 1 garlic cloves, minced (1 condiment)
- 1 (8-ounce) package button mushrooms, chopped (1 healthy fat)
- 2 cups low-sodium vegetable broth (2 condiments)
- ½ tsp. dried marjoram leaves (¼ green)
- ⅛ tsp. black pepper (¼ condiment)
- ⅔ cup grated Parmesan cheese (½ healthy fat)

Directions:

1. In a 6-quart slow cooker, mix the barley, garlic, mushrooms, broth, marjoram, and pepper.
2. Cover and cook on low for 7 to 8 hours, or until the barley has absorbed most of the liquid and is tender, and the vegetables are tender. Stir in the Parmesan cheese and serve.

Nutrition: Calories: 288; Fat: 6 g; Protein: 13 g.

227. Risotto with Green Beans and Sweet Potatoes

Serving: 4
Difficulty: 2
Preparation Time: 20 minutes
Cooking Time: 4 to 5 hours
Optavia Counts: 0 lean/ 1 green/ 4 healthy fat/ 2 condiments
Ingredients:

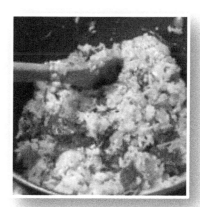

- 2 large sweet potato
- 2 garlic cloves, minced
- 2 cups short-grain brown rice
- 1 tsp. dried thyme leaves
- 6 cups low-sodium vegetable broth
- 2 cups green beans, cut in half crosswise
- 1 tbsp. unsalted butter
- ½ cup Parmesan cheese

Directions:

1. In a 6-quart slow cooker, mix the sweet potato, garlic, rice, thyme, and broth.
2. Cover and cook over low heat for 3 to 4 hours.
3. Mix in the green beans.
4. Cover and cook over low heat for 37 minutes.
5. Stir in the butter and cheese. Cover and cook at low for 20 minutes, then stir and serve.

Nutrition: Calories: 385; Fat: 10 g; Protein: 10 g.

228. Maple Lemon Tempeh Cubes

Serving: 4
Difficulty: 3
Preparation Time: 10 minutes
Cooking Time: 30 to 40 minutes
Optavia Counts: 0 lean/ 1 green/ 2 healthy fat/ 6 condiments
Ingredients:

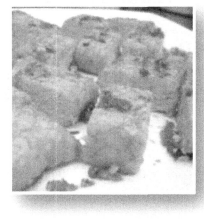

- 1 packet tempeh (½ healthy fat)
- 2 to 3 tsp. coconut oil (¼ healthy fat)
- 3 tbsp. lemon juice (¼ condiment)
- 2 tsp. maple syrup (¼ condiment)
- 1 to 2 tsp. Bragg's Liquid Aminos or low-sodium tamari or (optional) (¼ condiment)
- 2 tsp. water (¼ condiment)
- ¼ tsp. dried basil (¼ green)
- ¼ tsp. powdered garlic (¼ condiment)
- Black pepper (freshly grounded); to taste (¼ condiment)

Directions:

1. Heat your oven to 350°F.
2. Cut your tempeh block into squares in bite form.
3. Cook coconut oil at medium to high heat in a non-stick skillet.
4. When melted and heated, add the tempeh and cook on one side for 2-4 minutes, or until the tempeh turns down into a golden-brown color.
5. Flip the tempeh bits and cook for 2-4 minutes.
6. Mix the lemon juice, tamari, maple syrup, basil, water, garlic, and black pepper while tempeh is browning.
7. Drop the mixture over tempeh, then swirl to cover the tempeh.
8. Sauté for 2-3 minutes, then turn the tempeh and sauté 1-2 minutes more.
9. The tempeh, on both sides, should be soft and orange.

Nutrition: Carbohydrates: 22 g; Fats: 17 g; Protein: 21 g.

229. Quinoa with Vegetables

Serving: 4
Difficulty: 4
Preparation Time: 10 minutes
Cooking Time: 5 to 6 hours
Optavia Counts: 0 lean/ 3 green/ 1 healthy fat/ 4 condiments
Ingredients:

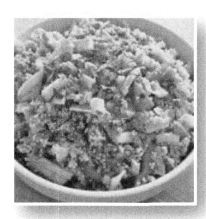

- 2/3 cups quinoa, rinsed and drained (1 healthy fat)
- 2 carrots, peeled and sliced (1 green)
- 1 pound cremini mushrooms (1 green)
- 3 garlic cloves, minced (¼ condiment)
- 2 cups low-sodium vegetable broth (1 condiment)
- ½ tsp. salt (¼ condiment)
- 1 tsp. dried marjoram leaves (¼ green)
- ⅛ tsp. black pepper (¼ condiment)

Directions:

1. In a 6-quart slow cooker, mix all of the ingredients.
2. Cook over low heat for 5 to 6 hours, covered.
3. Stir the mixture and serve.

Nutrition: Calories: 204; Fat: 3 g; Protein: 7 g.

CHAPTER 13.

SOUPS AND SALADS

230. Wasabi Tuna Asian Salad

Serving: 1
Difficulty: 1
Preparation Time: 30 minutes.
Cooking Time: 10 minutes.
Optavia Counts: 1 lean/ 2 green/ 1 healthy fat/ 4 condiments
Ingredients:

- 1 tsp. lime juice
- Non-stick cooking spray
- A dash of salt and pepper
- 1 tsp. wasabi paste
- 1 tsp. olive oil
- ½ cup chopped or shredded cucumbers
- 1 cup bok choy stalks
- 6 oz. raw tuna steak

Directions:
For the Fish:
1. Preheat your skillet to medium heat. Mix your wasabi and lime juice; coat the tuna steaks.
2. Use a non-stick cooking spray on your skillet for 10 seconds.
3. Put your tuna steaks on the skillet and cook over medium heat until you get the desired doneness.

For the Salad:
1. Slice the cucumber into match-stick tiny sizes. Cut the bok choy into minute pieces. Toss gently with pepper, salt, and olive oil if you want.

Nutrition: Calories: 380; Fiber: 1 g; Cholesterol: 115 mg; Saturated fat: 2 g; Protein: 61 g.

231. California Soup

Serving: 1
Difficulty: 1
Preparation Time: 10 minutes.
Cooking Time: 10 minutes.
Optavia Counts: 0 lean/ 0 green/ 1 healthy fat/ 1 condiments
Ingredients:

- 1 quart (960 ml) chicken broth, heated
- 1 large or 2 small, very ripe black avocados, pitted, peeled, and cut into chunks

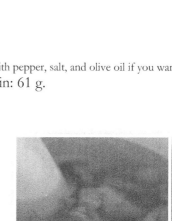

Directions:
1. Add the avocados with the broth in a blender puree until very smooth and serve.

Nutrition: Calories: 198; Fat: 11 g; Fiber: 1 g; Carbs: 12 g; Protein: 12 g.

232. Cheesy Cauliflower Soup

Serving: 1
Difficulty: 4
Preparation Time: 15 minutes
Cooking Time: 1 hour
Optavia Counts: 1 lean/ 4 green/ 2 healthy fat/ 5 condiments
Ingredients:

- 1 tbsp. minced scallion
- Bacon, cooked and drained
- Guar or xanthan (optional)
- ½ cups shredded cheddar cheese
- 1 ½ cups carb countdown dairy beverage or half-and-half
- 1 tsp. white vinegar - 1 tsp. salt
- 720 ml chicken broth - 1 tbsp. grated carrot
- 20 g. finely chopped celery
- 1 tbsp. finely chopped onion
- 600 g. cauliflower, diced small

Directions:

1. In a big, heavy-bottomed pan, place the cauliflower, onion, scallion, celery, and carrot. Add the broth, salt and vinegar to the chicken; bring it to a simmer and cook for about 30 to 45 minutes.
2. Stir in the carb countdown or half-and-half and then whisk in the cheese a bit at a time before adding more, allowing each additional time to melt. With guar or xanthan, thicken it a bit if you think it needs it. Cover each serving with slightly crumbled bacon and hazelnuts.

Nutrition: Calories: 270; Fat: 10 g; Protein: 10 g; Carbs: 10 g.

233. Egg Drop Soup

Serving: 1
Difficulty: 1
Preparation Time: 10 minutes.
Cooking Time: 10 minutes.
Optavia Counts: 1 lean/ 1 green/ 0 healthy fat/ 5 condiments
Ingredients:

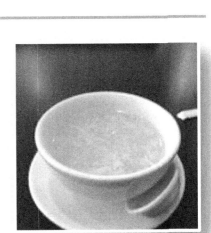

- 3 large eggs
- 2 scallion, sliced
- ½ tsp. grated fresh ginger
- 1 tbsp. rice vinegar
- 1 tbsp. soy sauce
- ¼ tsp. guar (optional)
- 1 quart chicken broth

Directions:

1. Put 1 cup or so of the chicken broth in your processor, turn it on medium and add the guar (if using). Let it mix for a moment and then put it in a big saucepan with the rest of the broth. (If you're not using the guar, then put all the liquid directly in a saucepan.) Put in the rice vinegar, soy sauce, ginger, and scallion. Heat over medium-high fire and let it boil for 5 to 10 minutes to let the flavors mix.
2. Beat the eggs in a glass mixing cup or small pitcher—something with a pouring edge. Using a fork to stir the soup surface in a gradual circle and pour in about ¼ of the eggs, stirring while cooking and turning them into shreds (which can occur almost instantly). Do three more times, using up half the egg.

Nutrition: Calories: 270; Fat: 10 g; Protein: 10 g; Carbs: 10 g.

234. Cauliflower, Spinach, and Cheese Soup

Serving: 1
Difficulty: 4
Preparation Time: 6 hours.
Cooking Time: 1 ½ hours.
Optavia Counts: 0 lean/ 2 green/ 2 healthy fat/ 8 condiments
Ingredients:

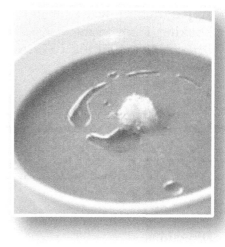

- 1 cup carb countdown dairy beverage
- Gouda cheese
- 675 g. shredded smoked
- cloves garlic, crushed
- ¼ tsp. pepper
- ½ tsp. salt or vega-sal
- ¼ tsp. cayenne
- 140 g. bagged baby spinach leaves, pre-washed
- ½ cup minced red onion
- 1 quart chicken broth
- Guar or xanthan
- 900 g. cauliflower florets, cut into ½-inch pieces

Directions:

1. Combine the broth, cauliflower, onion, spinach, cayenne, or vega-sal salt, pepper, and garlic in your slow cooker. Close the slow cooker, set it to low, and let simmer for 6 hours or until tender.
2. Stir in the gouda when the time's up, a little at a time, and then the carb timer. Cover the slow cooker again and steam for another 15 minutes or until the cheese has melted completely. Slightly thicken the broth with guar or xanthan.

Nutrition: Calories: 140; Fat: 3 g; Fiber: 2 g; Carbs: 1.5 g; Protein: 7 g.

235. Corner-Filling Soup

Serving: 1
Difficulty: 4
Preparation Time: ½ hour
Cooking Time: ½ hour
Optavia Counts: 0 lean/ 1 green/ 1 healthy fat/ 4 condiments
Ingredients:

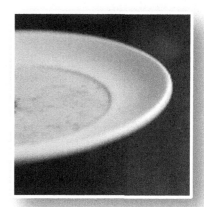

- ¼ tsp. pepper
- 30 ml. dry sherry
- 1 quart beef broth
- 1 small onion, sliced paper-thin
- 115 g. sliced mushrooms
- 28 g. butter

Directions:

1. In a pot, heat the butter and sauté the mushrooms and onions into the butter until they're soft.
2. Apply the broth, sherry, and pepper over the meat. For 5 to 10 minutes or so, let it steam, just to change the flavors a bit, and serve.

Nutrition: Carbs: 5.5 g; Fiber: 1.1 g; Protein: 8 g.

236. Lemon Greek Salad

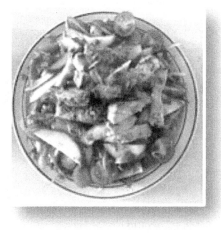

Serving: 2
Difficulty: 2
Preparation Time: 25 minutes
Cooking Time: 25 minutes
Optavia Counts: 1 lean/ 5 green/ 1 healthy fat/ 3 condiments
Ingredients:

- 140 oz. chicken breast
- 2 chopped cucumber
- 1 cup chopped orange/red bell pepper
- 1 cup wedged/sliced/chopped tomatoes
- ¼ cup chopped olives
- 1 tbsp. fresh parsley, finely chopped
- 1 tbsp. finely chopped red onion
- 1 tsp. lemon juice
- 1 tsp. olive oil
- 1 clove minced garlic

Directions:

1. Preheat your grill to medium heat. Grill the chicken and cook on each side until it is no longer pink or for 5 minutes. Cut the chicken into tiny pieces. In your serving bowl, mix garlic, olives, and parsley.
2. Whisk in 1 teaspoon of olive oil and 4 teaspoons of lemon juice. Add onion, tomatoes, bell pepper, and cucumber. Toss gently. Coat the ingredients with dressing. Add another teaspoon of lemon juice to taste. Divide the salad into two servings and put 6 oz. chicken on top of each salad.

Nutrition: Calories: 525; Fat: 47.4 g; Carbs: 9.3 g; Sugar: 3.8 g; Protein: 16.6 g; Cholesterol: 30 mg.

237. Peanut Soup

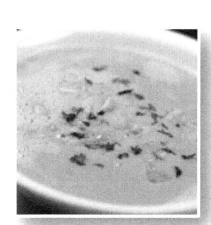

Serving: 2
Difficulty: 3
Preparation Time: 15 minutes
Cooking Time: 45 minutes
Optavia Counts: 0 lean/ 1 green/ 4 healthy fat/ 4 condiments
Ingredients:

- Salted peanuts, chopped
- 420 ml half-and-half or heavy cream
- 1 tsp. guar gum (optional
- 1 ¼ cups (325 g) natural peanut butter (Here, we used smooth)
- ½ tsp. salt or vega-sal
- l chicken broth
- 1 medium onion, finely chopped
- 2 ribs celery, finely chopped - 42 g. butter

Directions:

1. Melt the butter in a pot, then sauté the butter with the celery and onion. Stir in the broth, salt, and peanut butter. Cover and cook for at least 60 minutes at the lowest temperature, stirring now and then.
2. If you are using guar gum (without adding carbohydrates, it makes the soup thicker) scoop 1 cup of the soup out of the pot about 16 minutes before serving. To this cup, apply the guar gum, run the mixture for a couple of seconds through the blender and whisk it back into the broth.
3. Stir in half-and-a-half and cook for 15 minutes more. Connect the peanuts to the garnish.

Nutrition: Calories: 140; Fat: 3 g; Fiber: 2 g; Carbs: 1. 5 g; Protein: 7 g.

238. Artichoke Soup

Serving: 2
Difficulty: 3
Preparation Time: 15 minutes.
Cooking Time: 45 minutes.
Optavia Counts: 0 lean/ 1 green/ 1 healthy fat/ 8 condiments
Ingredients:

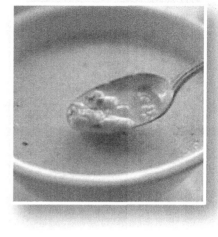

- Juice of ½ lemon
- ½ tsp. guar or xanthan
- 900 ml. chicken broth, divided
- 6 can quarter artichoke hearts, drained
- 1 clove garlic, crushed
- 1 stalk celery, finely chopped
- 1 small onion, finely chopped
- 1 tbsp. butter
- Salt or vega-sal - Pepper

Directions:

1. Melt the butter in a big skillet, then sauté the celery, onion, and garlic over low to medium heat. Shake from time to time. Drain the hearts of the artichoke and pick off any rough leaf pieces left on.
2. Place the heart of the artichoke in a food processor with the S-blade in place. Add ½ cup chicken broth and guar gum and strain until a fine purée is made from the artichokes. In a saucepan, scrape the artichoke mixture, add the remaining chicken broth, and boil over medium-high heat.
3. Stir the onion and celery into the artichoke mixture until tender. Whisk on the half-and-half when it comes to a boil. Take it back to a boil, push in the juice of a lemon and stir again. To taste, apply salt and pepper. You can eat this right now, hot, or you can eat it cooled in summers.

Nutrition: Fat: 12.0 g; Cholesterol: 101.9 mg; Sodium: 728.9 mg; Carbs: 11.9 g; Fiber: 1.9 g.

239. Curried Pumpkin Soup

Serving: 2
Difficulty: 3
Preparation Time: 30 minutes.
Cooking Time: 30 minutes.
Optavia Counts: 0 lean/ 0 green/ 1 healthy fat/ 7 condiments
Ingredients:

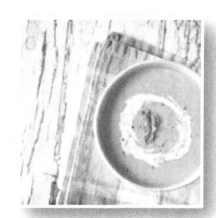

- 1 tsp. curry powder
- ½ cup carb countdown dairy beverage
- 1 ½ cups canned pumpkin
- 4 cups chicken broth
- 1 tbsp. butter
- 1 clove garlic
- ¼ cup minced onion
- Salt and pepper to taste

Directions:

1. In a big saucepan, sauté the garlic and onion in butter, heavy-bottomed saucepan with medium-low heat until only softened. Put in the broth of the chicken and cook for half an hour. Mix in the dairy beverage carb countdown, canned pumpkin, and curry powder. Adjust to a boil and cook softly for a further 15 minutes. To taste, incorporate salt and pepper, and then eat.

Nutrition: Fat: 12.0 g; Cholesterol: 101.9 mg; Sodium: 728.9 mg; Carbs: 11.9 g; Fiber: 1.9 g.

240. Cheesy Onion Soup

Serving: 2
Difficulty: 4
Preparation Time: 1 hour.
Cooking Time: 1 hour.
Optavia Counts: 0 lean/ 0 green/ 3 healthy fat/ 4 condiments
Ingredients:

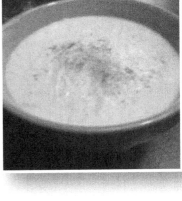

- ½ cup carb countdown dairy beverage
- Medium onion
- 1 quart beef broth
- ½ cup heavy cream
- Guar or xanthan (optional)
- 1 ½ cups shredded sharp cheddar cheese
- Salt and pepper to taste

Directions:

1. In a large saucepan, add the beef broth and start heating it over a medium-high flame. Cut the paper-thin onion and apply it to the broth. Switch the heat down to low as the broth begins to boil and let the entire thing steam for 1 hour. You should do this ahead of time if you like; turn off the heat, let the entire thing cool, refrigerate it, and later do the rest. If you do this, before moving, lift the broth from heating again. Stir in the cream and the dairy beverage carb timer softly. Now stir in the cheese, a little at a time, until all of it has melted in. If you want to thicken with guar or xanthan, stir with a ladle or spoon instead of a whisk, you don't want to sever the onion threads.
2. Garnish with salt and pepper and serve.

Nutrition: Fat: 12.0 g; Cholesterol: 101.9 mg; Sodium: 728.9 mg; Carbs: 11.9 g; Fiber: 1.9 g.

241. Cream of Potato Soup

Serving: 2
Difficulty: 5
Preparation Time: 1 hour
Cooking Time: 5 hours
Optavia Counts: 0 lean/ 2 green/ 1 healthy fat/ 4 condiments
Ingredients:

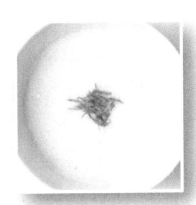

- ½ cup carb countdown dairy beverage
- ½ cup heavy cream - ½ cup ketones mix
- ½ cup chopped onion
- ½ head cauliflower, chunked
- 1 quart chicken broth guar or xanthan (optional)
- 1 bunch Scallions, sliced

Directions:

1. In your slow cooker, put cauliflower, broth, and onion. Close and set the slow cooker to low and run for about 4 to 5 hours. We use a hand mixer to purée the soup right in the slow cooker; so alternatively, you should pass the cauliflower and onion into your blender or food processor, along with 1 cup of broth. Purée until entirely smooth, and then blend into the ketones, either way. If the cauliflower has been withdrawn from the slow cooker for purée, add the purée back in and whisk it back into the remaining broth. Stir in the carb countdown and cream. If you believe it needs it, thicken it a little more with guar or xanthan.
2. To taste, apply salt and pepper and mix in the sliced scallions. Serve instantly hot or chill and serve as Vichyssoise.

Nutrition: Fat: 12.0 g; Cholesterol: 101.9 mg; Sodium: 728.9 mg; Carbs: 11.9 g; Fiber: 1.9 g.

242. Swiss Cheese and Broccoli Soup

Serving: 3
Difficulty: 4
Preparation Time: 10 minutes
Cooking Time: 1 hour
Optavia Counts: 0 lean/ 1 green/ 4 healthy fat/ 3 condiments
Ingredients:

- Guar or xanthan
- 360 g. shredded Swiss cheese
- 1 cup heavy cream
- 500 ml carb countdown dairy beverage
- 10 oz. frozen chopped broccoli, thawed
- 28 oz. chicken broth
- 28 g. butter - 420 g. minced onion

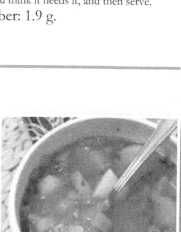

Directions:

1. Sauté the onion into the butter in a big, heavy-bottomed saucepan until it is transparent. Put the broccoli and the chicken broth in the pan and cook for 20 to 30 minutes until the broccoli is very soft.
2. Mix in the countdown carb and some cream. Brought it to a simmer again. Now mix in the cheese, a little at a time, allowing each batch to melt before adding any more. Thicken a bit with guar or xanthan when all the cheese is melted if you think it needs it, and then serve.

Nutrition: Fat: 12.0 g; Cholesterol: 101.9 mg; Sodium: 728.9 mg; Carbs: 11.9 g; Fiber: 1.9 g.

243. Tavern Soup

Serving: 3
Difficulty: 4
Preparation Time: 8 to 10 hours
Cooking Time: 1 hour
Servings: 8
Optavia Counts: 0 lean/ 4 green/ 1 healthy fat/ 7 condiments
Ingredients:

- ½ tsp. hot pepper sauce
- ½ tsp. salt or vega-sal - 24 oz. light beer
- 900 g. sharp cheddar cheese, shredded
- 1 tsp. pepper - ½ cup chopped fresh parsley
- ½ cup shredded carrot
- ½ cup finely diced green bell pepper
- ½ cup finely diced celery
- Guar or xanthan - l chicken broth

Directions:

1. Mix in your slow cooker celery, broth, green pepper, parsley, and pepper. Close the slow cooker, set it to low, and let it steam for 6 to 8 hours (it won't hurt for a little longer). To purée the vegetables in the slow cooker right there until the time is up, use a handheld blender to scoop them out with a slotted spoon, and purée them in the blender, then add them to the slow cooker.
2. Now swirl a little at a time in the cheese until it's all melted. Add the hot pepper sauce, beer, salt, or vega-sal, and mix until the foaming ends. To thicken the broth, use guar or xanthan until it is about sour cream thickness. Cover the pot again, turn it too heavy, and simmer for an additional 20 minutes before eating.

Nutrition: Fat: 12.0 g; Cholesterol: 101.9 mg; Sodium: 728.9 mg; Carbs: 11.9 g; Fiber: 1.9 g.

244. Broccoli Blue Cheese Soup

Serving: 3
Difficulty: 4
Preparation Time: 1 hour.
Cooking Time: 1 hour.
Optavia Counts: 0 lean/ 2 green/ 4 healthy fat/ 2 condiments
Ingredients:

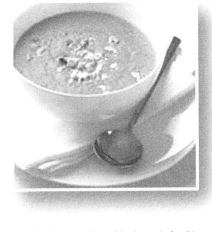

- 1 cup crumbled blue cheese
- ¼ cup heavy cream
- 1 pound frozen broccoli, thawed
- 1 ½ quarts chicken broth
- 1 cup carb countdown dairy beverage
- 1 turnip, peeled and diced
- 28 g. butter - 160 g. chopped onion

Directions:

1. Sauté the onion in the butter over medium-low heat in a broad saucepan—you don't want it to tan.
2. Until the onion is soft and transparent, add the chicken broth and the turnip to your pot. Brought the blend to a boil and let it cook for 20 to 30 minutes over medium to low heat.
3. Put in the thawed broccoli and cook for the next 20 minutes. With a slotted spoon, spoon the vegetables out and put them in a Mixer. A ladleful broth is added to the mix, and the blender runs until the vegetables are finely puréed. Shift the mixture back to your pot. Stir in the carb countdown, the heavy cream, and the blue cheese. Simmer for the next 5 to 10 minutes stirring periodically, and serve.

Nutrition: Fat: 12.0 g; Cholesterol: 101.9 mg; Sodium: 728.9 mg; Carbs: 11.9 g; Fiber: 1.9 g.

245. Cream of Mushroom Soup

Serving: 3
Difficulty: 5
Preparation Time: 6 hours
Cooking Time: 1 ½ hours
Servings: 5 or 7
Optavia Counts: 0 lean/ 1 green/ 1 healthy fat/ 5 condiments
Ingredients:

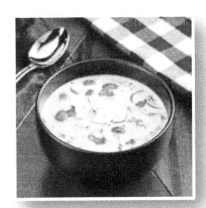

- ½ cup light sour cream
- ½ cup heavy cream
- 1 quart chicken broth
- 28 g. butter
- ¼ cup chopped onion
- 225 g. mushrooms, sliced
- Guar or xanthan (optional)

Directions:

1. Sauté the onion and mushrooms in the butter in a large, heavy skillet until the mushrooms soften and change color. Move them to a slow cooker. Put in the broth. Cover your slow cooker, set it Low and let it cook for 5 to 6 hours. Scrape the vegetables with a slotted spoon when the time is up, and stick them in your blender or any food processor. Add in enough broth to help them quickly process and finely purée them. Put the puréed vegetables back into the slow cooker, using a rubber scraper to clean out any last piece. Now whisk in the heavy cream and sour cream and apply to taste the salt and pepper. If you think it deserves it, thicken the sauce a little with guar or xanthan. Serve asp.

Nutrition: Calories: 525; Fat: 47.4 g; Carbs: 9.3 g; Sugar: 3.8 g; Protein: 16.6 g; Cholesterol: 30 mg.

246. Healthy Broccoli Salad

Serving: 3
Difficulty: 2
Preparation Time: 5 minutes
Cooking Time: 25 minutes
Optavia Counts: 1 lean/ 1 green/ 1 healthy fat/ 4 condiments
Ingredients:

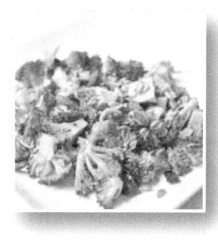

- 8 cups broccoli, chopped
- 1 tbsp. apple cider vinegar
- ½ cup Greek yogurt
- 1 tbsp. sunflower seeds
- 3 Bacon slices, cooked and chopped
- 1 cup onion, sliced
- ¼ tsp. stevia

Directions:

1. In a mixing bowl, mix broccoli, onion, and bacon.
2. In a small bowl, mix yogurt, vinegar, and stevia and pour over the broccoli mixture.
3. Stir to combine.
4. Sprinkle sunflower seeds on top of the salad.
5. Store salad in the refrigerator for 30 minutes.
6. Serve and enjoy.

Nutrition: Calories: 90; Fat: 4.9 g; Carbs: 5.4 g; Sugar: 2.5 g; Protein: 6.2 g; Cholesterol: 12 mg.

247. Olive Soup

Serving: 3
Difficulty: 4
Preparation Time: 20 minutes
Cooking Time: 1 hour
Optavia Counts: 0 lean/ 0 green/ 1 healthy fat/ 6 condiments
Ingredients:

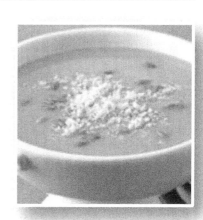

- Pepper
- Salt or vega-sal
- ¼ cup dry sherry
- ½ tsp. guar or xanthan
- 1 cup minced black olives. (You can buy cans of minced black olives)
- 1 cup heavy cream
- 4 cups chicken broth, divided

Directions:

1. Put ½ cup of the chicken broth with the guar gum in the blender and pulse for a few moments.
   Pour the remainder of the stock and the olives into a saucepan and add the blended mixture.
2. Heat and then whisk in the cream before simmering. Return to a boil, stir in the sherry, then apply salt and pepper to taste.

Nutrition: Carbs: 3.5 g; Fiber: 1.1 g; Protein: 2.5 g.

248. Salmon Soup

Serving: 4
Difficulty: 2
Preparation Time: 15 minutes.
Cooking Time: 21 minutes.
Optavia Counts: 1 lean/ 4 green/ 1 healthy fat/ 3 condiments
Ingredients:

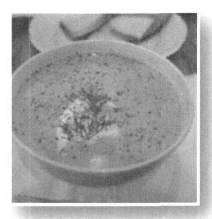

- 1 pound salmon fillets
- 1 tbsp. olive oil
- 1 cup carrots, peeled and chopped
- ½ cup celery stalk, chopped
- ¼ cup yellow onion, chopped
- 1 cup cauliflower, chopped
- 5 cups chicken broth
- Salt and ground black pepper, as required
- ¼ cup fresh parsley, chopped

Directions:

1. Arrange a steamer trivet in the lower part of the Instant Pot and pour 1 cup of water. Place the salmon fillets on top of the trivet in a single layer. Secure the lid and switch to the role of "Seal".
2. Cook on "Manual" with "High Pressure" for about 7 to 8 minutes. Press "Cancel" and carefully do a "Quick" release.
3. Remove the lid and transfer the salmon onto a plate. Cut the salmon into bite-sized pieces.
4. Remove the water and trivet from Instant Pot.
5. Add the oil in Instant Pot and select "Sauté". Then add the carrot, celery, and onion and cook for about 5 minutes or until browned completely. Press "Cancel" and stir in the cauliflower and broth. Secure the lid and switch to the role of "Seal".
6. Cook on "Manual" with "High Pressure" for about 8 minutes. Press "Cancel" and do a "Natural" release.
7. Remove the lid and stir in salmon pieces and black pepper until well combined.
8. Serve immediately with the garnishing of parsley.

Nutrition: Calories: 525; Fat: 47.4 g; Carbs: 9.3 g; Sugar: 3.8 g; Protein: 16.6 g; Cholesterol: 30 mg.

249. Loaded Potato Soup

Serving: 4
Difficulty: 3
Preparation Time: 15 minutes
Cooking Time: 30 minutes
Optavia Counts: 1 lean/ 2 green/ 1 healthy fat/ 7 condiments
Ingredients:

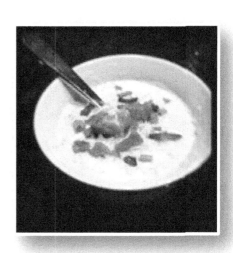

- 1 package (12 oz) bacon, chopped
- 1 ½ cups onion, chopped
- 2 garlic cloves, minced
- 2 pounds russet potatoes, peeled and chopped
- 6 cups chicken broth
- 4 cups whole milk
- ½ tsp. sea salt
- ½ tsp. freshly ground black pepper
- 1 ½ cups shredded cheddar cheese
- Sour cream, for serving (optional)
- Chopped fresh chives, for serving (optional)

Directions:

1. Preheat for 5 minutes.
2. Add the bacon, onion, and garlic. Cook, stirring occasionally, for 5 minutes. Set aside some of the bacon for garnish. Add the potatoes and chicken broth. Set pressure lid, making sure the pressure release valve is in the seal position. Select pressure and set it too high. Set time to 10 minutes, then select start/stop to begin. At the point when pressure cooking is finished, fast deliver the pressure by moving the weight discharge valve to the vent position. Cautiously eliminate top when the unit has got done with delivering pressure.
3. Add the milk and mash the ingredients until the soup reaches your desired consistency. Season with salt and black pepper. Sprinkle the cheese evenly over the top of the soup. Close crisping lid. Select broil and set the time to 5 minutes. Select start/stop to begin.
4. When cooking is complete, top with the reserved crispy bacon and serve with sour cream and chives (if using).

Nutrition: Calories: 468; Total fat: 19 g; Saturated fat: 9 g; Cholesterol: 51 mg; Sodium: 1041 mg; Carbs: 53 g; Fiber: 8 g; Protein: 23 g.

250. Butternut Squash, Apple, Bacon and Orzo Soup

Serving: 4
Difficulty: 2
Preparation Time: 10 minutes
Cooking Time: 28 minutes
Optavia Counts: 1 lean/ 2 green/ 1 healthy fat/ 3 condiments
Ingredients:

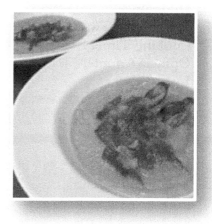

- 2 slices uncooked bacon, cut into ½-inch pieces
- 12 oz. butternut squash, peeled and cubed
- 1 green apple, cut into small cubes
- Kosher salt
- Freshly ground black pepper
- 1 tbsp. minced fresh oregano
- 2 quarts chicken stock
- 1 cup orzo

Directions:

1. Select sear/sauté and set the temperature to High. Select start/stop to begin. Let preheat for 5 minutes.
2. Set the bacon in the pot and cook, stirring frequently, about 5 minutes, or until fat is rendered and the bacon starts to brown. Using a slotted spoon, bring the bacon to a paper towel-lined plate to drain, leaving the rendered bacon fat in the pot.
3. Add the butternut squash, apple, salt, and pepper and sauté until partially soft, about 5 minutes. Stir in the oregano.
4. Attach the bacon back into the pot along with the chicken stock. Bring to a boil for about 10 minutes, then add the orzo. Cook for about 8 minutes, until the orzo is tender. Serve.

Nutrition: Calories: 247; Total fat: 7 g; Saturated fat: 2 g; Cholesterol: 17 mg; Sodium: 563 mg; Carbs: 33 g; Fiber: 3 g; Protein: 12 g.

251. Chicken Enchilada Soup

Serving: 4
Difficulty: 2
Preparation Time: 5 minutes.
Cooking Time: 30 minutes.
Optavia Counts: 1 lean/ 1 green/ 1 healthy fat/ 7 condiments
Ingredients:

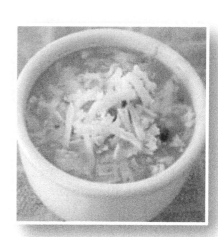

- 1 tbsp. extra-virgin olive oil
- 1 small red onion, diced
- 1 (14 oz) cans fire-roasted tomatoes with chilies
- 1 can corn
- 1 can black beans, rinsed and drained
- 1 can red enchilada sauce
- 1 can tomato paste
- 1 tbsp. taco seasoning
- 1 tbsp. freshly squeezed lime juice
- 1 pound boneless, skinless chicken breasts
- Salt
- Freshly ground black pepper

Directions:

1. Select sear/sauté and set the temperature to High. Select start/stop to begin. Let preheat for 5 minutes.
2. Place the olive oil and onion in the pot. Cook until the onions are translucent, about 2 minutes.
3. Add the tomatoes, corn, beans, enchilada sauce, tomato paste, taco seasoning, lime juice, and chicken. Season with salt and pepper and stir. Set pressure lid, making sure the pressure release valve is in the seal position.
4. Select pressure and set it to High. Set time to 9 minutes. Select start/stop to begin.
5. When pressure cooking is processed, allow pressure to release naturally for 10 of the vent position. Carefully remove the cover when the unit has finished releasing pressure.
6. Bring the chicken breasts to a cutting board. Using two forks, shred the chicken. Return the chicken back to the pot and stir. Serve in a bowl with toppings of choice, such as shredded cheese, crushed tortilla chips, sliced avocado, sour cream, cilantro, and lime wedges, if desired.

Nutrition: Calories: 257; Total Fat: 4 g; Saturated Fat: 0 g; Cholesterol: 33 mg; Sodium: 819 mg; Carbs: 37 g; Fiber: 7 g; Protein: 20 g.

252. Tex-Mex Chicken Tortilla Soup

Serving: 4
Difficulty: 2
Preparation Time: 10 minutes
Cooking Time: 20 minutes
Optavia Counts: 1 lean/ 1 green/ 1 healthy fat/ 11 condiments
Ingredients:

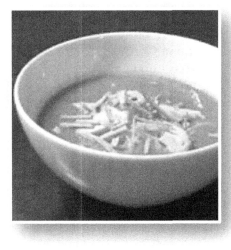

- 1 tbsp. extra-virgin olive oil
- 1 onion, chopped
- 1 pound boneless, skinless chicken breasts
- 2 cups chicken broth
- 1 jar salsa
- 3 tbsp. tomato paste
- 1 tbsp. chili powder
- 1 tsp. cumin
- ½ tsp. sea salt
- ½ tsp. freshly ground black pepper
- 1 pinch of cayenne pepper
- 1 can black beans, rinsed and drained
- 1 ½ cups frozen corn
- Tortilla strips, for garnish

Directions:

1. Select sear/sauté and set to temperature to High. Select start/stop to begin. Let preheat for 5 minutes.
2. Place the olive oil and onions into the pot and cook, stirring occasionally, for 5 minutes.
3. Add the chicken breast, chicken broth, salsa, tomato paste, chili powder, cumin, salt, pepper, and cayenne pepper. Set pressure lid, making sure the pressure release valve is in the seal position.
4. When pressure cooking is complete, allow pressure to release naturally for 10 minutes. After 10 minutes, quickly relieve residual pressure by moving the pressure relief valve to the vent position. Carefully remove the cover when the unit has finished releasing pressure.
5. Bring the chicken breasts to a cutting board and shred with two forks. Set aside.
6. Add the black beans and corn. Select sear/sauté and set to md. Select start/stop to begin. Cook until heated through, about 5 minutes.
7. Add shredded chicken back to the pot. Garnish with tortilla strips, serve, and enjoy!

Nutrition: Calories: 186; Total Fat: 4 g; Saturated Fat: 0 g; Cholesterol: 33 mg; Sodium: 783 mg; Carbs: 23 g; Fiber: 6 g; Protein: 19 g.

253. White Bean and Cabbage Soup

Serving: 4
Difficulty: 2
Preparation Time: 5 minutes
Cooking Time: 30 minutes
Optavia Counts: 1 lean/ 4 green/ 1 healthy fat/ 3 condiments
Ingredients:

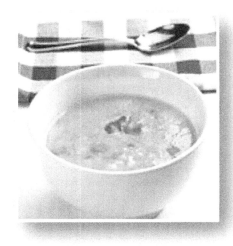

- 1 tbsp. olive oil
- 2 medium carrots
- 4 stalks of celery or 1 chopped bok choy
- 1 onion
- 4 cloves minced garlic
- 1 chopped cabbage head
- ½ pound northern beans soaked in water overnight
- 2 cups chicken broth
- 1 quart water

Directions:

1. Whisk vegetables in oil.
2. Attach the rest of the ingredients and cook on medium-low heat for 30 minutes.

Nutrition: Calories: 423; Fat: 2 g; Fiber: 0 g; Carbs: 20 g; Protein: 33 g.

CHAPTER 14.

DESSERT RECIPES

254. Yogurt Mint

Serving: 1
Difficulty: 1
Preparation Time: 5 minutes
Cooking Time: 10 minutes
Optavia Counts: 0 lean/ 1 green/ 2 healthy fat/ 1 condiments
Ingredients:

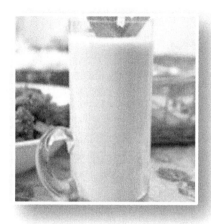

- 1 cup water
- 1 cup milk
- ¾ cup plain yogurt
- ¼ cup fresh mint
- 1 tbsp. maple syrup

Directions:

1. Put 1 cup of water into the Instant Pot Pressure Cooker.
2. Press the "Steam" function button and adjust to 1 minute.
3. Once done, add the milk, then press the "Yogurt" function button and allow boiling.
4. Add yogurt and fresh mint, then stir well. Pour into a glass and add maple syrup. Enjoy.

Nutrition: Calories: 25; Fat: 0.5 g; Carbs: 5 g; Protein: 2 g.

255. Rice Pudding

Serving: 1
Difficulty: 1
Preparation Time: 5 minutes
Cooking Time: 12 minutes
Optavia Counts: 0 lean/ 0 green/ 1 healthy fat/ 5 condiments
Ingredients:

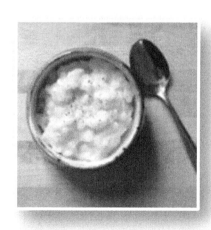

- ½ cup short grain rice
- ¼ cup sugar
- Cinnamon stick
- ½ cup milk
- 1 slice lemon peel
- Salt to taste

Directions:

1. Rinse the rice under cold water.
2. Put the milk, cinnamon stick, sugar, salt, and lemon peel inside the Instant Pot Pressure Cooker.
3. Close the lid and make sure to seal the valve. Press the "Pressure" button and cook for 10 minutes on High. When the timer beeps, choose the "Quick Pressure" release. This will take about 2 minutes.
4. Remove the lid. Open the pressure cooker and discard the lemon peel and cinnamon stick. Spoon in a serving container and serve.

Nutrition: Calories: 111; Fat: 6 g; Carbs: 21 g; Protein: 3 g.

256. Braised Apples

Serving: 1
Difficulty: 1
Preparation Time: 5 minutes
Cooking Time: 12 minutes
Optavia Counts: 0 lean/ 0 green/ 0 healthy fat/ 3 condiments
Ingredients:

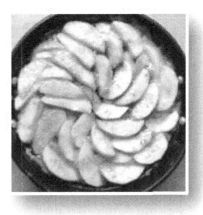

- 4 cored apples
- ½ cup water
- ½ cup red wine
- 1 tbsp. sugar
- ½ tsp. ground cinnamon

Directions:

1. In the bottom of an Instant Pot, add the water and place apples.
2. Pour wine on top and sprinkle with sugar and cinnamon. Close the lid carefully and cook for 10 minutes at high pressure.
3. When done, do a quick pressure release.
4. Transfer the apples onto serving plates and top with cooking liquid.
5. Serve immediately.

Nutrition: Calories: 245; Fat: 0.5 g; Carbs: 11 g; Protein: 1 g.

257. Wine Figs

Serving: 1
Difficulty: 1
Preparation Time: 5 minutes
Cooking Time: 3 minutes
Optavia Counts: 0 lean/ 1 green/ 1 healthy fat/ 2 condiments
Ingredients:

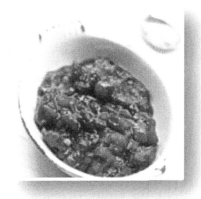

- ½ cup pine nuts
- 1 cup red wine
- 1 pound figs
- Sugar, as needed

Directions:

1. Slowly pour the wine and sugar into the Instant Pot.
2. Arrange the trivet inside it; place the figs over it. Close the lid and lock. Ensure that you have sealed the valve to avoid leakage.
3. Press "Manual" mode and set the timer to 3 minutes.
4. After the timer reads zero, press "Cancel" and "Quick Pressure."
5. Carefully remove the lid.
6. Divide figs into containers, and sprinkle wine from the pot over them.
7. Top with pine nuts and enjoy.

Nutrition: Calories: 94; Fat: 3 g; Carbs: 5 g; Protein: 2 g.

258. Cinnamon Bites

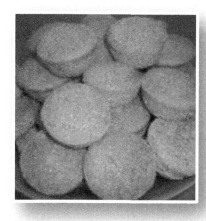

Serving: 1
Difficulty: 4
Preparation Time: 20 minutes
Cooking Time: 95 minutes
Optavia Counts: 0 lean/ 0 green/ 3 healthy fat/ 4 condiments
Ingredients:

- ⅛ tsp. nutmeg
- 1 tsp. vanilla extract
- ¼ tsp. cinnamon
- 1 tbsp. coconut oil
- ½ cup butter, grass-fed
- 16 oz. cream cheese
- Stevia to taste

Directions:

1. Soften your coconut oil and butter, mixing in your cream cheese.
2. Add all of your remaining ingredients, and mix well.
3. Pour into molds, and freeze until set.

Nutrition: Calories: 178; Protein: 1 g; Fat: 19 g.

259. Sweet Chai Bites

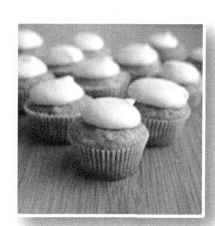

Serving: 2
Difficulty: 3
Preparation Time: 20 minutes
Cooking Time: 45 minutes
Optavia Counts: 0 lean/ 0 green/ 2 healthy fat/ 8 condiments
Ingredients:

- 8 oz 225gr cream cheese
- 2 tsp. coconut oil
- ¾ cup butter, grass-fed
- 1 tsp. ginger
- 1 tsp. cardamom
- 1 tsp. nutmeg
- 1 tsp. cloves
- 1 tsp. vanilla extract, pure
- 1 tsp. Darjeeling black tea
- Stevia to taste

Directions:

1. Melt your coconut oil and butter before adding in your black tea. Allow it to sit for 1–2 minutes.
2. Add in your cream cheese, removing your mixture from heat.
3. Add in all of your spices, and stir to combine.
4. Pour into molds, and freeze before serving.

Nutrition: Calories: 178; Protein: 1 g; Fat: 19 g.

260. Lemon Curd

Serving: 2
Difficulty: 1
Preparation Time: 10 minutes
Cooking Time: 10 minutes
Optavia Counts: 1 lean/ 0 green/ 1 healthy fat/ 4 condiments
Ingredients:

- 1 tbsp. butter
- 2/3 cup sugar
- ⅔ cup lemon juice
- 2 eggs
- 1 tsp. lemon zest
- 1 ½ cup water

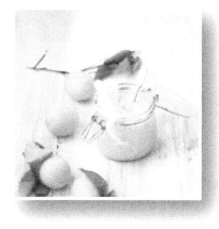

Directions:

1. Beat the sugar and butter thoroughly until it is smooth.
2. Add 2 whole eggs and incorporate just the yolk of the other egg.
3. Add the lemon juice.
4. Transfer the mixture into the 2 jars and tightly seal the tops.
5. Pour 1 ½ cups water into the bottom of the Instant Pot and place in a steaming rack. Put the jars on the rack and cook on high pressure for 10 minutes.
6. Natural-release the pressure for 10 minutes before quickly releasing the rest.
7. Stir in the zest and put the lids back on the jars.

Nutrition: Calories: 45; Fat: 1 g; Carbs: 8 g; Protein: 1 g.

261. Rhubarb Dessert

Serving: 2
Difficulty: 1
Preparation Time: 4 minutes
Cooking Time: 5 minutes
Optavia Counts: 0 lean/ 1 green/ 1 healthy fat/ 2 condiments
Ingredients:

- 3 cups rhubarb, chopped
- 1 tbsp. ghee, melted
- ⅓ cup water
- 1 tbsp. stevia
- 1 tsp. vanilla extract

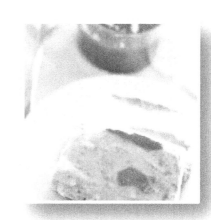

Directions:

1. Put all the listed ingredients in your Instant Pot, cover, and cook on high for 5 minutes.
2. Divide into small containers and serve cold.
3. Enjoy!

Nutrition: Calories: 83; Fat: 2 g; Carbs: 2 g; Protein: 2 g.

262. Raspberry Compote

Serving: 2
Difficulty: 2
Preparation Time: 11 minutes
Cooking Time: 30 minutes
Optavia Counts: 0 lean/ 0 green/ 0 healthy fat/ 4 condiments
Ingredients:

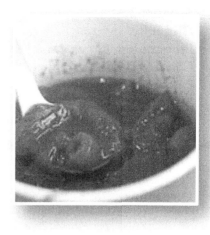

- 2 pints raspberries
- ½ cup Swerve
- 1 tsp. freshly grated lemon zest
- 1 tsp. vanilla extract
- 1 cup water

Directions:

1. Press the cook button on your Instant Pot, add all the listed ingredients.
2. Turn well and pour in 1 cup water.
3. Cook for 5 minutes, continually stirring. Then pour in additional 1 cup water and press the "Cancel" button.
4. Secure the lid properly, press the "Manual" button, and set the timer to 15 minutes on low pressure.
5. When the timer buzzes, press the "Cancel" button and release the pressure naturally for 10 minutes.
6. Move the pressure handle to the "Venting" position to release any remaining pressure and open the lid.
7. Let it cool before serving.

Nutrition: Calories: 48; Fat: 0.5 g; Carbs: 5 g; Protein: 1 g.

263. Poached Pears

Serving: 2
Difficulty: 1
Preparation Time: 8 minutes
Cooking Time: 10 minutes
Optavia Counts: 0 lean/ 1 green/ 0 healthy fat/ 4 condiments
Ingredients:

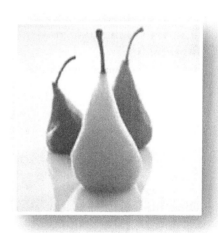

- 1 tbsp. lime juice
- 1 tsp. lime zest
- 1 x 7cm cinnamon stick
- 4 whole pears, peeled
- 1 cup water
- Fresh mint leaves for garnish

Directions:

1. Add all components: except for the mint leaves to the Instant Pot.
2. Seal the Instant Pot and choose the "Manual" button.
3. Cook on high for 10 minutes.
4. Perform a natural pressure release.
5. Remove the pears from the pot.
6. Serve in containers and garnish with mint on top.

Nutrition: Calories: 59; Fat: 0.1 g; Carbs: 14 g; Protein: 0.3 g.

264. Apple Crisp

Serving: 2
Difficulty: 1
Preparation Time: 10 minutes
Cooking Time: 13 minutes
Optavia Counts: 0 lean/ 0 green/ 0 healthy fat/ 3 condiments
Ingredients:

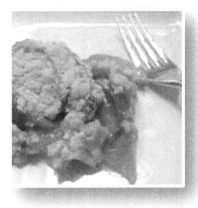

- 6 cups apples, sliced into chunks
- 1 tsp. cinnamon
- ¼ cup rolled oats
- ¼ cup brown sugar
- ½ cup water

Directions:

1. Put all the listed ingredients in the pot and mix well.
2. Seal the pot, choose "Manual" mode, and cook at high pressure for 8 minutes.
3. Release the pressure naturally and let sit for 5 minutes or until the sauce has thickened.
4. Serve and enjoy.

Nutrition: Calories: 218; Fat: 5 g; Carbs: 5 g; Protein: 2 g.

265. Tasty Banana Cake

Serving: 3
Difficulty: 2
Preparation Time: 10 minutes
Cooking Time: 30 minutes
Optavia Counts: 1 lean/ 0 green/ 3 healthy fat/ 4 condiments
Ingredients:

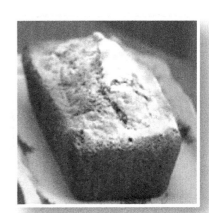

- ½ cup butter, soft
- 2 eggs
- ⅓ cup brown sugar
- 1 tbsp. honey
- 1 banana
- 1 cup white flour
- 1 tbsp. baking powder
- ½ tbsp. cinnamon powder
- Cooking spray

Directions:

1. Spray cake skillet with cooking spray.
2. Add in butter with egg, sugar, banana, cinnamon, honey, flour, and baking powder in a container then beat.
3. Pour batter into cake pan filled with cooking spray, place in a deep fryer, and cook at 350°F for 30 minutes.
4. Let cool, cut into slices.
5. Serve.

Nutrition: Calories: 435; Fat: 7 g; Carbs: 15 g; Protein: 2 g.

266. Mini Lava Cakes

Serving: 3
Difficulty: 2
Preparation Time: 5 minutes
Cooking Time: 20 minutes
Optavia Counts: 1 lean/ 0 green/ 2 healthy fat/ 5 condiments
Ingredients:

- 2 large eggs
- 2 tbsps. sugar
- 4 tbsps. olive oil
- ¼ cup milk
- 1 tsp. flour
- 1/8 cup cocoa powder
- ½ tbsp. baking powder
- ½ tbsp. orange zest

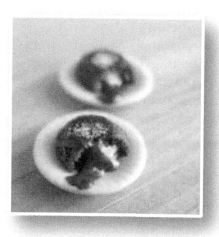

Directions:

1. Mix in egg with sugar, flour, salt, oil, milk, orange zest, baking powder, and cocoa powder, turn properly. Move it to oiled ramekins.
2. Put ramekins in an Air Fryer and cook at 320°F for 20 minutes.
3. Serve warm.

Nutrition: Calories: 329; Fat: 8.5 g; Carbs: 12.1 Protein: 4 g.

267. Apple Bread

Serving: 3
Difficulty: 3
Preparation Time: 5 minutes
Cooking Time: 40 minutes
Optavia Counts: 1 lean/ 0 green/ 2 healthy fat/ 5 condiments
Ingredients:

- 3 cup apples
- 1 cup sugar
- 1 tbsp. vanilla
- 2 eggs
- 1 tbsp. apple pie spice
- 2 cup white flour
- 1 tbsp. baking powder
- 1 stick butter
- 1 cup water

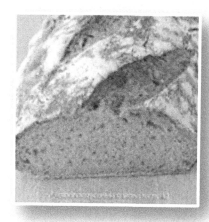

Directions:

1. Mix in egg with 1 butter stick, sugar, and apple pie spice and turn using a mixer.
2. Put apples and turn properly.
3. Mix baking powder with flour in another container and turn.
4. Blend the 2 mixtures, turn and move them to the spring-form skillet.
5. Get the spring-form skillet into an Air Fryer and cook at 320°F for 40 minutes
6. Slice. Serve.

Nutrition: Calories: 401; Fat: 9 g; Carbs: 19 g; Protein: 3 g.

268. Chocolate Orange Bites

Serving: 3
Difficulty: 4
Preparation Time: 20 minutes
Cooking Time: 120 minutes
Optavia Counts: 0 lean/ 0 green/ 1 healthy fat/ 3 condiments
Ingredients:

- 10 oz. coconut oil
- 1 tbsp. cocoa powder
- ¼ tsp. orange extract
- Stevia to taste

Directions:

1. Melt half of your coconut oil using a double boiler, and then add in your stevia and orange extract.
2. Get out candy molds, pouring the mixture into them. Fill each mold halfway, and then place them in the fridge until they are set.
3. Melt the other half of the coconut oil, stirring in your cocoa powder and stevia, making sure that the mixture is smooth with no lumps.
4. Pour into your molds, filling them up all the way, and then allow them to set in the fridge before serving.

Nutrition: Calories: 188; Protein: 1 g; Fat: 21 g; Carbs: 5 g.

269. Caramel Cones

Serving: 3
Difficulty: 4
Preparation Time: 25 minutes
Cooking Time: 120 minutes
Optavia Counts: 0 lean/ 0 green/ 1 healthy fat/ 6 condiments
Ingredients:

- 2 cups heavy whipping cream
- 2 tbsps. sour cream
- 1 tbsp. caramel sugar
- 1 tsp. sea salt, fine
- ⅓ cup butter, grass-fed
- ⅓ cup coconut oil
- Stevia to taste

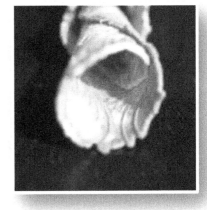

Directions:

1. Soften the coconut oil and butter, mixing.
2. Mix all ingredients to form a batter, and then place them in molds.
3. Top with a little salt, and keep refrigerated until serving.

Nutrition: Calories: 100; Fat: 12 g; Carbs: 1 g.

270. Chocolate Fondue

Serving: 3
Difficulty: 1
Preparation Time: 5 minutes
Cooking Time: 10 minutes
Optavia Counts: 0 lean/ 0 green/ 1 healthy fat/ 2 condiments
Ingredients:

- 1 cup water
- ½ tsp. sugar
- ½ cup coconut cream
- ¾ cup dark chocolate, chopped

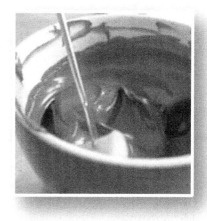

Directions:

1 Pour the water into your Instant Pot.
2 To a heatproof bowl, add the chocolate, sugar, and coconut cream.
3 Place in the Instant Pot.
4 Seal the lid, select MANUAL, and cook for 2 minutes. When ready, do a quick release and carefully open the lid. Stir well and serve immediately.

Nutrition: Calories: 216; Fat: 17 g; Carbs: 11 g; Protein: 2 g.

271. Banana Bread

Serving: 3
Difficulty: 3
Preparation Time: 5 minutes
Cooking Time: 40 minutes
Optavia Counts: 1 lean/ 0 green/ 3 healthy fat/ 6 condiments
Ingredients:

- ¾ cup sugar
- ⅓ cup butter
- 1 tbsp. vanilla extract
- 1 egg
- 3 ripe bananas
- 1 tbsp. baking powder
- 1 ½ cup flour
- ½ tbsp. baking soda
- ⅓ cup milk
- 1 ½ tbsp. cream of tartar
- Cooking spray

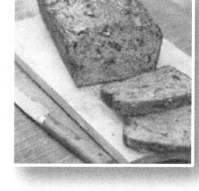

Directions:

1. Mix in milk with cream of tartar, vanilla, egg, sugar, bananas, and butter in a container and turn whole.
2. Mix in flour with baking soda and baking powder.
3. Blend the 2 mixtures, turn properly and move into oiled skillet with cooking spray. Put into the Air Fryer, and cook at 320°F for 40 minutes.
4. Remove bread, allow to cool, slice.
5. Serve.

Nutrition: Calories: 25; Fat: 16 g; Carbs: 18 g; Protein: 13 g.

272. Bread Pudding

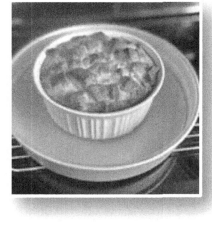

Serving: 4
Difficulty: 2
Preparation Time: 10 minutes
Cooking Time: 10 minutes
Optavia Counts: 1 lean/ 0 green/ 1 healthy fat/ 2 condiments
Ingredients:
- 1 doz. glazed doughnuts
- 2 cups cherries
- 6 egg yolks
- ½ cup whipping cream
- ½ cup raisins
- ¼ cup sugar
- ½ cup chocolate chips

Directions:
1. Add cherries with whipping cream and egg in a container then turn properly.
2. Combine in raisins with chocolate chips, doughnuts, and sugar in a container, then stir.
3. Mix the 2 mixtures, pour into the oiled skillet then into the Air Fryer and cook at 310°F for 1 hour.
4. Cool pudding before cutting.
5. Serve.

Nutrition: Calories: 456; Fat: 11 g; Carbs: 6 g; Protein: 12 g.

273. Wrapped Pears

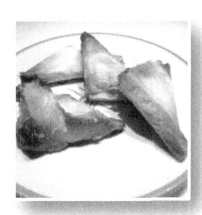

Serving: 4
Difficulty: 1
Preparation Time: 10 minutes
Cooking Time: 10 minutes
Optavia Counts: 1 lean/ 0 green/ 1 healthy fat/ 2 condiments
Ingredients:
- 1 puff pastry sheets
- 14 oz. vanilla custard
- 2 pears
- 1 egg
- ½ tbsp. cinnamon powder
- 4 cups sugar

Directions:
1. Put wisp pastry slices on a flat surface, add a spoonful of vanilla custard at the middle of each, add pear halves and wrap.
2. Sweep pears with egg and cinnamon. Spray sugar, put into Air Fryer's basket, and cook at 320°F for 15 minutes.
3. Split parcels on plates.
4. Serve.

Nutrition: Calories: 285; Fat: 14 g; Carbs: 13 Protein: 45 g.

274. Cocoa Cake

Serving: 4
Difficulty: 1
Preparation Time: 5 minutes
Cooking Time: 17 minutes
Optavia Counts: 1 lean/ 0 green/ 1 healthy fat/ 4 condiments
Ingredients:

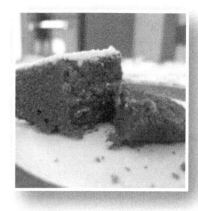

- 1 tbsp. butter
- 2 eggs
- 2 cups sugar
- ¾ cup cocoa powder
- 2 cups flour
- ½ tbsp. lemon juice

Directions:

1. Combine 1 tbsp. butter with cocoa powder in a container and beat.
2. Mix in the rest of the butter with eggs, flour, sugar, and lemon juice in another container, blend properly and move half into a cake skillet.
3. Add half of the cocoa blend, spread, add the rest of the butter layer, and crest with the remaining cocoa.
4. Put into an Air Fryer and cook at 360°F for 17 minutes.
5. Allow the cooling before slicing.
6. Serve.

Nutrition: Calories: 221; Fat: 5 g; Carbs: 12 g; Protein: 13 g.

275. Fluffy Bites

Serving: 4
Difficulty: 4
Preparation Time: 20 minutes
Cooking Time: 60 minutes
Optavia Counts: 1 lean/ 1 green/ 0 healthy fat/ 5 condiments
Ingredients:

- 1 tsp. cinnamon
- ⅔ cup sour cream
- 2 cups heavy cream
- 1 tsp. scraped vanilla bean
- ¼ tsp. cardamom
- 6 egg yolks
- Stevia to taste

Directions:

1. Start by whisking your egg yolks until creamy and smooth.
2. Get out a double boiler, and add your eggs with the rest of the ingredients. Mix well.
3. Remove from heat, allowing it to cool until it reaches room temperature.
4. Refrigerate for 1 hour before whisking well.
5. Pour into molds, and freeze for at least an hour before serving.

Nutrition: Calories: 363; Protein: 2 g; Fat: 40 g; Carbs: 1 g.

276. Strawberry Cheesecake Minis

Serving: 4
Difficulty: 5
Preparation Time: 30 minutes
Cooking Time: 120 minutes
Optavia Counts: 0 lean/ 0 green/ 2 healthy fat/ 3 condiments
Ingredients:

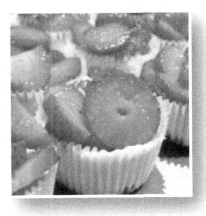

- 1 cup coconut oil
- 1 cup coconut butter
- ½ cup strawberries, sliced
- ½ tsp. lime juice
- 1 tbsp. cream cheese, full fat
- Stevia to taste

Directions:

1. Blend the strawberries.
2. Soften the cream cheese, and then add in the coconut butter.
3. Combine all ingredients, and then pour the mixture into silicone molds.
4. Freeze for at least 2 hours before serving.

Nutrition: Calories: 372; Protein: 1 g; Fat: 41 g; Carbs: 2 g.

CHAPTER 15.

FUELING HACKS RECIPES

277. Berry Mojito

Serving: 1
Difficulty: 1
Preparation Time: 10 minutes
Cooking Time: 0 minutes
Optavia Counts: 0 lean/ 1 green/ 0 healthy fat/ 1 condiments
Ingredients:

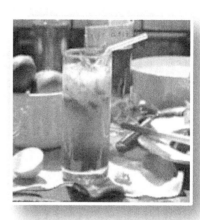

- 1 cup water
- ½ sachet Essential1 Mixed Berry Flavor Infuser
- 3 fresh mint leaves
- 1 tbsp. fresh lime juice
- Ice cubes, as required

Directions:

1. Take a cocktail glass and put the lime juice and mint leaves in the bottom.
2. With the bottom end of a spoon, gently muddle the mint leaves.
3. Add the Berry Infuser and water to the glass and stir to combine.
4. Add ice cubes.
5. Serve and enjoy!

Serving Suggestion: Garnish it with a wedge of lime and some mint leaves.
Variation Tip: You can use frozen berries instead of fresh ones.
Nutrition Per serving: Calories: 26; Fat: 0.3 g; Sat Fat: 0.1 g; Carbs: 6.6 g; Fiber: 2.5 g; Sugar: 0.7 g; Protein: 1.3 g.

278. Vanilla Frappé

Serving: 1
Difficulty: 1
Preparation Time: 5 minutes
Cooking Time: 0 minutes
Optavia Counts: 0 lean/ 0 green/ 3 healthy fat/ 0 condiments
Ingredients:

- ½ cup ice
- 2 tbsp. whipped topping
- ½ cup unsweetened almond milk
- 1 sachet Essential Creamy Vanilla Shake

Directions:

1. Put the shake mixture, almond milk, and ice into a blender.
2. Blend until smooth. Pour the mixture into a glass.
3. Top it with the whipped topping. Serve and enjoy!

Serving Suggestion: You can add cherries or berries as a pretty garnish.
Variation Tip: Use coconut syrup for a tropical flavor.
Nutrition Per serving: Calories: 308; Fat: 11.2 g; Sat Fat: 1.5 g; Carbs: 10.4 g; Fiber: 9 g; Sugar: 2.2 g; Protein: 41.1 g.

279. Vanilla Shake

Serving: 1
Difficulty: 1
Preparation Time: 5 minutes
Cooking Time: 0 minutes
Optavia Counts: 0 lean/ 0 green/ 1 healthy fat/ 1 condiments
Ingredients:

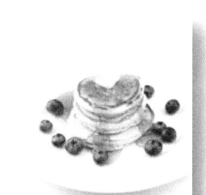

- 10 oz. water
- ½ sachet Essential Creamy Vanilla Shake
- ½ cup unsweetened almond milk
- 1 tsp. Essential Spiced Gingerbread
- 12 ice cubes

Directions:

1. Place all the ingredients in a blender and pulse until smooth.
2. Pour the drink into serving glasses and serve.

Serving Suggestion: Garnish with whipped cream, a morello cherry, and a sprinkling of chocolate shavings.
Variation Tip: You can use vanilla ice cream to prepare a thicker milkshake.
Nutrition Per serving: Calories: 130; Fat: 3.3 g; Sat Fat: 0.2 g; Carbs: 15 g; Fiber: 4.5 g; Sugar: 6 g; Protein: 13 g.

280. Maple Pancakes

Serving: 1
Difficulty: 1
Preparation Time: 10 minutes
Cooking Time: 6 minutes
Optavia Counts: 1 lean/ 1 green/ 1 healthy fat/ 2 condiments
Ingredients:

- ¼ cup water
- ¼ tsp. ground cinnamon
- 1 sachet stevia
- 1 tbsp. Egg Beaters
- ¼ tsp. baking powder
- 1 sachet Essential Old-Fashioned Maple & Brown Sugar Oatmeal
- 1 tbsp. sugar-free pancake syrup

Directions:

1. Add all the ingredients (except for the syrup) to a large bowl.
2. Combine them until well mixed.
3. Gently grease a skillet and warm it on medium-high.
4. Add a few tablespoons of the mixture to the skillet and cook on both sides until golden brown. Repeat until all the mixture is used.
5. Drizzle with the pancake syrup before serving.

Serving Suggestion: Serve with a topping of pomegranate seeds or blueberries.
Variation Tip: You can also add some vanilla extract to enhance the flavor.
Nutrition Per serving: Calories: 11; Fat: 2.5 g; Sat Fat: 0.5 g; Carbs: 33.2 g; Fiber: 3.3 g; Sugar: 9.1 g; Protein: 5.9 g.

281. Brownie Pudding Cups

Serving: 1
Difficulty: 1
Preparation Time: 10 minutes
Cooking Time: 1 minute
Servings: 2
Optavia Counts: 0 lean/ 0 green/ 0 healthy fat/ 1 condiments
Ingredients:

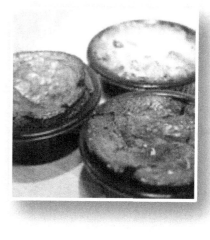

- 2 Sachets Essential Chocolate Fudge Pudding
- 1 tbsp. sugar-free caramel syrup
- 1 cup water, divided
- 2 sachets Essential Decadent Chocolate Brownie

Directions:

1. In a bowl, add the brownie mix and 3 tablespoons of water and combine well.
2. Divide the mixture equally into ramekins and microwave each for 1 minute.
3. Chill the mixtures completely.
4. In a bowl, add the pudding mix to the remaining water, and mix well.
5. Divide the pudding mixture over the brownie mixture equally.
6. Drizzle each mixture with the caramel syrup, and with a knife, swirl the caramel into pudding.
7. Refrigerate until set completely.

Serving Suggestion: Top with crushed Oreos before serving.
Variation Tip: You can use sugar-free chocolate syrup if you prefer.
Nutrition Per serving: Calories: 106; Fat: 2.1 g; Sat Fat: 0.4 g; Carbs: 21.8 g; Fiber: 0.5 g; Sugar: 0 g; Protein: 0.6 g.

282. Tiramisu Shake

Serving: 2
Difficulty: 1
Preparation Time: 5 minutes
Cooking Time: 0 minutes
Optavia Counts: 0 lean/ 0 green/ 0 healthy fat/ 1 condiments
Ingredients:

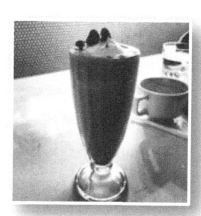

- 1 cup water
- 1 cup ice, crushed
- 2 tbsp. sugar-free chocolate syrup
- 2 sachets Essential Frothy Cappuccino Boost

Directions:

1. Place all the ingredients into a blender and pulse until smooth and creamy.
2. Pour the shake into a serving glass.
3. Serve and enjoy!

Serving Suggestion: You can serve with chocolate syrup, ladyfinger cookies, and whipped cream on top.
Variation Tip: You can add some vanilla extract to the shake.
Nutrition Per serving: Calories: 106; Fat: 3 g; Sat Fat: 1 g; Carbs: 17 g; Fiber: 0 g; Sugar: 10 g; Protein: 1 g.

283. Potato Bagels

Serving: 2
Difficulty: 1
Preparation Time: 15 minutes
Cooking Time: 12 minutes
Optavia Counts: 1 lean/ 1 green/ 1 healthy fat/ 0 condiments

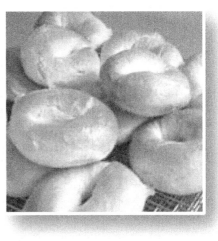

Ingredients:

- 2 egg whites
- 2 tbsp. baking powder
- 2 Sachets Essential Roasted Garlic Creamy Smashed Potatoes

Directions:

1. Preheat the oven to 350°F.
2. Lightly grease the holes of a donut pan.
3. Take a bowl, add the egg whites and beat until foamy.
4. Add the baking powder and mashed potatoes mixture and beat until well blended.
5. Place the mixture into the prepared donut holes.
6. Bake for 10 to 12 minutes (or until completely baked through).
7. Serve warm.

Serving Suggestion: Serve warm with some cream cheese.

Variation Tip: You can sprinkle on seeds or seasoning of your choice before baking and broil the bagels after cooking for extra crispiness.

Nutrition Per serving: Calories: 106; Fat: 1.1 g; Sat Fat: 0.4 g; Carbs: 15.7 g; Fiber: 0.1 g; Sugar: 0.5 g; Protein: 9.1 g.

284. Tropical Smoothie Bowl

Serving: 2
Difficulty: 1
Preparation Time: 10 minutes
Cooking Time: 0 minutes
Optavia Counts: 0 lean/ 0 green/ 1 healthy fat/ 3 condiments

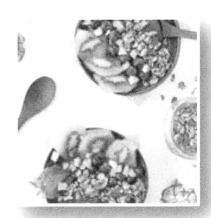

Ingredients:

- 2 tbsp. unsweetened coconut, shredded
- 1 tsp. chia seeds
- 1 tsp. lime zest, grated
- 2 tbsp. cashews
- 1 cup ice cubes
- 1 cup unsweetened coconut milk
- 1 sachet Essential Tropical Fruit Smoothie

Directions:

1. Put the smoothie mixture, coconut milk, and ice cubes into a blender and pulse until smooth.
2. Take a serving bowl and add the mixture to it.
3. Top with the remaining ingredients.
4. Serve and enjoy!

Serving Suggestion: Add a variety of toppings such as berries, toasted coconut, or seeds.

Variation Tip: You can also add chocolate syrup to sweeten the bowl further.

Nutrition Per serving: Calories: 944; Fat: 41.2 g; Sat Fat: 28.6 g; Carbs: 142.1 g; Fiber: 12.5 g; Sugar: 103.1 g; Protein: 8.5 g.

285. Mocha Cake

Serving: 2
Difficulty: 1
Preparation Time: 5 minutes
Cooking Time: 2 minutes
Optavia Counts: 1 lean/ 1 green/ 1 healthy fat/ 0 condiments
Ingredients:

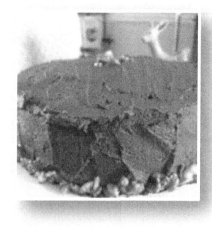

- ¼ cup water
- ¼ tsp. baking powder
- 1 tbsp. egg beaters
- 1 sachet stevia
- 1 sachet Essential Golden Chocolate Chip Pancakes
- 1 sachet Essential Frothy Cappuccino Boost

Directions:

1. Add all of the ingredients to a microwave-safe bowl and stir until they are well combined.
2. Place the mixture into the microwave for 1 to 2 minutes.
3. Take the cake out from the microwave and cut it in half horizontally.
4. Serve warm.

Serving Suggestion: Layer with sugar-free frosting and top with a few cacao nibs for some crunch.
Variation Tip: This cake is perfect as it is!
Nutrition Per serving: Calories: 195; Fat: 4.5 g; Sat Fat: 1 g; Carbs: 28.9 g; Fiber: 2.5 g; Sugar: 11 g; Protein: 11 g.

286. Little Fudge Balls

Serving: 2
Difficulty: 1
Preparation Time: 10 minutes
Cooking Time: 0 minutes
Optavia Counts: 0 lean/ 0 green/ 2 healthy fat/ 0 condiments
Ingredients:

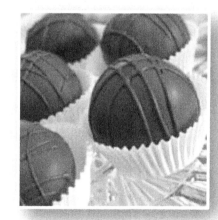

- 1 tbsp. powdered peanut butter
- ¼ cup unsweetened almond milk
- 1 tbsp. water
- 1 Sachet Essential Creamy Chocolate shake
- 1 Sachet Essential Chocolate Fudge Pudding

Directions:

1. Add all the ingredients to a small bowl and blend until well combined.
2. Make eight little equal-sized balls from the mixture.
3. Place the balls onto a parchment paper-lined baking sheet and refrigerate until set.

Serving Suggestion: Serve with chocolate sprinkles on top.
Variation Tip: You can use coconut milk instead of almond.
Nutrition Per serving: Calories: 538; Fat: 14.3 g; Sat Fat: 7.2 g; Carbs: 81.8 g; Fiber: 5.8 g; Sugar: 57.5 g; Protein: 24.5 g.

287. Brownie Cookies

Serving: 2
Difficulty: 1
Preparation Time: 10 minutes
Cooking Time: 2 minutes 20 seconds
Optavia Counts: 0 lean/ 0 green/ 0 healthy fat/ 0 condiments
Ingredients:

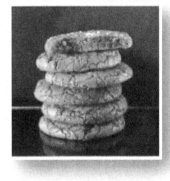

- ⅓ cup water
- 2 Sachets Essential Decadent Chocolate Brownie
- 1 Essential Silky Peanut Butter & Chocolate Chip Bar

Directions:

1. In a bowl, add the brownie mix and water; mix well. Set aside.
2. Put the peanut butter and chocolate bar in a microwave-safe bowl and microwave on High for 20 seconds or until slightly melted.
3. Add the crunch bar to the brownie mixture and mix until well combined.
4. Divide the mixture into 2 small microwave-safe ramekins and microwave on high for 2 minutes.
5. Remove from the microwave and set aside to cool for 5 minutes before serving.
6. Enjoy!

Serving Suggestion: Top with your favorite type of nuts or chocolate chips.
Variation Tip: You can also add milk chocolate or white chocolate chunks to the mixture.
Nutrition Per serving: Calories: 186; Fat: 6.1 g; Sat Fat: 2.1 g; Carbs: 25.8 g; Fiber: 2 g; Sugar: 6 g; Protein: 8.6 g.

288. Zucchini Spaghetti

Serving: 2
Difficulty: 1
Preparation Time: 20 minutes
Cooking Time: 15 minutes
Optavia Counts: 0 lean/ 2 green/ 2 healthy fat/ 3 condiments
Ingredients:

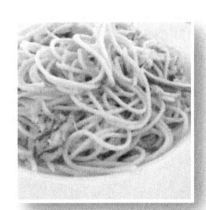

- 1 pound zucchinis, cut with a spiralizer
- 1 cup Parmesan, grated
- ¼ cup parsley, chopped.
- ¼ cup olive oil
- 1 garlic cloves; minced
- ½ tsp. red pepper flakes
- Salt and black pepper to taste.

Directions:

1. In a pan that fits into your Air Fryer, mix all the ingredients, toss, put into the fryer and cook at 370°F for 15 minutes.
2. Divide between plates and serve as a side dish.

Nutrition: Calories: 200; Fat: 6 g; Carbs: 4 g; Protein: 5 g.

289. Cabbage and Radishes Mix

Serving: 3
Difficulty: 1
Preparation Time: 20 minutes
Cooking Time: 15 minutes
Optavia Counts: 0 lean/ 3 green/ 1 healthy fat/ 4 condiments
Ingredients:

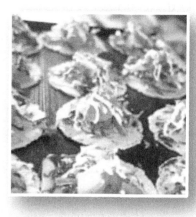

- ½ small head green cabbage; shredded
- ½ cup celery leaves; chopped.
- ¼ cup green onions; chopped.
- 1 bunch radishes; sliced
- 1 tbsp. olive oil
- 2 tbsps. balsamic vinegar
- ½ tsp. hot paprika
- 1 tsp. lemon juice

Directions:

1. In your Air Fryer pan, combine all the ingredients and toss well.
2. Place the pan in the fryer and cook at 380°F for 15 minutes. Divide between plates and serve as a side dish.

Nutrition: Calories: 130; Fat: 4 g; Carbs: 4 g; Protein: 7 g.

290. Flavorsome Waffles

Serving: 3
Difficulty: 1
Preparation Time: 18 minutes
Cooking Time: 8 minutes
Optavia Counts: 0 lean/ 0 green/ 0 healthy fat/ 3 condiments
Ingredients:

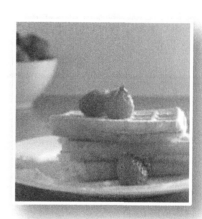

- ½ cup water
- 1 tbsp. canned pumpkin
- ½ tsp. pumpkin pie spice
- 2 Sachets Essential Golden Chocolate Chip Pancakes
- 1 tbsp. sugar-free pancake syrup

Directions:

1. Grease and preheat the waffle iron.
2. Place all the ingredients in a bowl, except for the pancake syrup, and blend until well combined.
3. Place half of the mixture into the preheated waffle iron and cook for 3 to 4 minutes or until golden brown.
4. Repeat with the remaining mixture.
5. Serve warm!

Serving Suggestion: Drizzle the waffle with pancake syrup.
Variation Tip: Add chopped strawberries or cherries on top for an even yummier taste.
Nutrition Per serving: Calories: 139; Fat: 4.6 g; Sat Fat: 1 g; Carbs: 21.8 g; Fiber: 0.8 g; Sugar: 6.3 g; Protein: 3.1 g.

291. Richly Tasty Crepe

Serving: 3
Difficulty: 1
Preparation Time: 10 minutes
Cooking Time: 4 minutes
Optavia Counts: 0 lean/ 1 green/ 1 healthy fat/ 2 condiments
Ingredients:

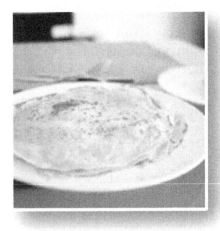

- ⅛ tsp. vanilla extract
- 1 tbsp. sugar-free chocolate syrup
- 1 tsp. stevia
- ¼ cup part-skim ricotta cheese
- ¼ cup water
- 1 sachet Essential Golden Chocolate Chip Pancakes

Directions:

1. Put the pancake mix and water in a bowl and blend well.
2. Heat a lightly greased frying pan over medium fire.
3. Pour the mixture into the pan and swirl it around to create a thin, round crepe.
4. Cook for 1 to 2 minutes on each side or until golden brown.
5. Place the crepe on a plate and carefully cut a slit in the middle.
6. Put the cheese, stevia, and vanilla extract in a small bowl and blend until well combined.
7. Place the mixture inside the crepe.
8. Serve and enjoy!

Serving Suggestion: Drizzle with chocolate syrup.
Variation Tip: Add chopped hazelnuts to the cheese mixture to enhance the flavor of the crepe.
Nutrition Per serving: Calories: 365; Fat: 13.9 g; Sat Fat: 5.1 g; Carbs: 47.3 g; Fiber: 1.1 g; Sugar: 13.9 g; Protein: 13.1 g.

292. Crunchy Cookies

Serving: 3
Difficulty: 1
Preparation Time: 10 minutes
Cooking Time: 15 minutes
Optavia Counts: 0 lean/ 1 green/ 1 healthy fat/ 2 condiments
Ingredients:

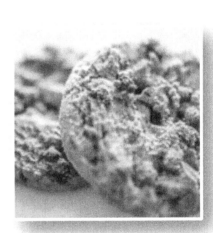

- 1 sachet stevia
- ½ tsp. vanilla extract
- ⅛ tsp. baking powder
- ⅓ cup water
- ⅛ tsp. ground cinnamon
- 1 Sachet Essential Old-Fashioned Maple & Brown Sugar Oatmeal
- 1 Essential Raisin Oat Cinnamon Crisp Bar

Directions:

1. Preheat the oven to 350°F. Line a cookie sheet with parchment paper.
2. Put the crisp bar in a microwave-safe bowl and microwave on High for 15 seconds or until it has melted slightly.
3. Gradually add the remaining ingredients to the bowl and mix until well combined. Set the mixture aside for 5 minutes.
4. Using a spoon, place four cookies onto the cookie sheet and lightly press down on each with your fingers.
5. Bake for 12 to 15 minutes or until golden brown.
6. Remove the cookie sheet from the oven and place it onto a wire rack to cool for 5 minutes.
7. Turn out the cookies onto the wire rack to cool before serving.

Serving Suggestion: Serve with chocolate chips on top.
Variation Tip: You can use brown sugar for extra sweetness.
Nutrition Per serving: Calories: 110; Fat: 2.1 g; Sat Fat: 0.9 g; Carbs: 16 g; Fiber: 3.4 g; Sugar: 2.8 g; Protein: 7.3 g.

293. Delicious French Toast Sticks

Serving: 3
Difficulty: 1
Preparation Time: 15 minutes
Cooking Time: 4 minutes
Optavia Counts: 1 lean/ 0 green/ 1 healthy fat/ 1 condiments
Ingredients:

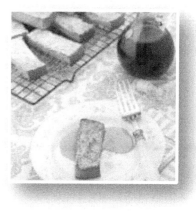

- 2 tbsp. low-fat cream cheese, softened
- Cooking spray
- 6 tbsp. liquid egg substitute
- 2 sachets Essential Cinnamon Crunchy O's Cereal

Directions:

1. Put the cereal in a food processor and pulse to a fine breadcrumb-like consistency.
2. Add the liquid egg substitute and cheese and pulse until a dough is formed.
3. Divide the dough into six parts and form these into toast stick shapes.
4. Heat a lightly greased pan over medium-high fire and cook the toast sticks for 2 minutes on each side or until golden brown.
5. Serve warm.

Serving Suggestion: Top with icing sugar before serving.
Variation Tip: You can add some honey to enhance the flavor.
Nutrition Per serving: Calories: 120; Fat: 3 g; Sat Fat: 1.5 g; Carbs: 17.7 g; Fiber: 1.3 g; Sugar: 5.6 g; Protein: 6.4 g.

294. Shamrock Shake

Serving: 3
Difficulty: 1
Preparation Time: 5 minutes
Cooking Time: 0 minutes
Optavia Counts: 0 lean/ 0 green/ 2 healthy fat/ 2 condiments
Ingredients:

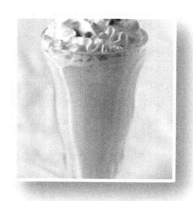

- ¼ tsp. peppermint extract
- 10 drops green food coloring
- 1 cup ice cube, crushed
- ¾ cup unsweetened almond milk
- 1 sachet Essential Creamy Vanilla Shake

Directions:

1. Place all the ingredients in a blender and pulse until smooth. Transfer the shake into a serving glass and serve immediately. Serving Suggestion: Top the shake with whipped cream, green sprinkles, and morello cherry. Variation Tip: Add an extra hint of vanilla extract to the shake for an enhanced taste.

Nutrition Per serving: Calories: 250; Fat: 10.9 g; Sat Fat: 1.2 g; Carbs: 30.5 g; Fiber: 3.7 g; Sugar: 7.1 g; Protein: 10.7 g.

295. Pumpkin Waffles

Serving: 4
Difficulty: 1
Preparation Time: 10 minutes
Cooking Time: 8 minutes
Optavia Counts: 0 lean/ 0 green/ 0 healthy fat/ 4 condiments
Ingredients:

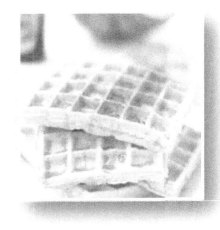

- 1 cup water
- Pinch of ground cinnamon
- 1 tsp. pumpkin pie spice
- 1 tbsp. canned pumpkin
- 2 sachets Essential Golden Pancake mixture
- 1 tbsp. sugar-free pancake syrup

Directions:

1. Lightly grease and heat the waffle iron.
2. In a bowl, add all the ingredients except the syrup and blend until well combined.
3. Place half the mixture into the preheated waffle iron and cook for 3 to 4 minutes or until golden brown.
4. Repeat with the remaining mixture.
5. Serve the waffles warm and drizzled with the pancake syrup. Enjoy!

Serving Suggestion: Serve with some toasted pumpkin seeds.
Variation Tip: You can use honey instead of pancake syrup.
Nutrition Per serving: Calories: 148; Fat: 3.1 g; Sat Fat: 0.3 g; Carbs: 27.5 g; Fiber: 3.2 g; Sugar: 11.4 g; Protein: 3.6 g.

296. Chocolate Donuts

Serving: 4
Difficulty: 1
Preparation Time: 5 minutes
Cooking Time: 15 minutes
Optavia Counts: 1 lean/ 0 green/ 2 healthy fat/ 1 condiments
Ingredients:

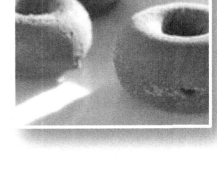

- ½ tsp. vanilla extract
- ½ tsp. baking powder
- ¼ cup unsweetened almond milk
- 1 tbsp. liquid egg substitute
- 2 Sachets Essential Golden Chocolate Chip Pancakes
- 2 Sachets Essential Decadent Chocolate Brownie

Directions:

1. Preheat the oven to 350°F. Lightly grease 4 holes of a donut pan.
2. Take a bowl, add all the ingredients, and mix until well blended.
3. Evenly place the mixture into the prepared donut pan.
4. Bake for 12 to 15 minutes or until the donuts are set completely.
5. Remove from the oven and set aside to cool slightly before eating.

Serving Suggestion: Serve with chocolate chips or crushed Oreos on top.
Variation Tip: You can use any other kind of milk.
Nutrition Per serving: Calories: 212; Fat: 7.2 g; Sat Fat: 1.5 g; Carbs: 31.1 g; Fiber: 1.6 g; Sugar: 11.2 g; Protein: 6.4 g.

297. Chicken Nuggets

Serving: 4
Difficulty: 1
Preparation Time: 10 minutes
Cooking Time: 20 minutes
Optavia Counts: 2 lean/ 0 green/ 1 healthy fat/ 2 condiments
Ingredients:

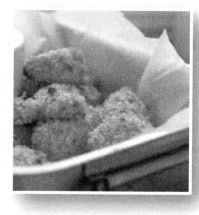

- 1 tbsp. olive oil
- 1 large egg
- 1 tbsp. Essential Honey Mustard & Onion Sticks, finely crushed
- ¾ pound boneless, skinless chicken breast, cubed
- 1 tbsp. lemon juice

Directions:

1. Preheat the oven to 400°F. Line a baking sheet with a lightly greased piece of foil.
2. Crack the egg into a bowl and beat it well. Place the crushed sticks into another bowl.
3. Dip the chicken cubes in the beaten egg mixture and then coat with the crushed sticks.
4. Arrange the coated chicken cubes onto the prepared baking sheet in a single layer and coat with cooking spray. Bake for 18 to 20 minutes, flipping once halfway through.
5. Remove the baking sheet from the oven and set the nuggets aside to cool slightly.

Serving Suggestion: Serve with ketchup (or any of your favorite sauces!).
Variation Tip: You can add any kind of seasonings according to your taste.
Nutrition Per serving: Calories: 134; Fat: 3.4 g; Sat Fat: 0.4 g; Carbs: 4.6 g; Fiber: 0.8 g; Sugar: 2.3 g; Protein: 19.9 g.

298. Peanut Butter Cookies

Serving: 4
Difficulty: 1
Preparation Time: 10 minutes
Cooking Time: 15 minutes
Optavia Counts: 0 lean/ 0 green/ 3 healthy fat/ 2 condiments
Ingredients:

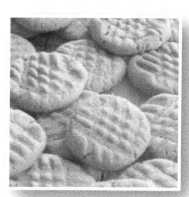

- ¼ tsp. vanilla extract
- ⅛ tsp. sea salt
- 1 tbsp. margarine, softened
- ¼ cup unsweetened almond milk
- ¼ tsp. baking powder
- 2 Sachets Essential Silky Peanut Butter Shake

Directions:

1. Heat the oven to 350°F. Take a bowl and add the shake mixture and baking powder and blend well.
2. Add the almond milk, margarine, and vanilla and combine well.
3. Mold the cookie dough into balls and place them onto a lined cookie sheet in a single layer.
4. Using a fork, lightly press each ball and sprinkle with some salt.
5. Place the cookie sheet into the oven and cook for 15 minutes.
6. Take the cookie sheet out of the oven and allow it to cool for 5 minutes. Turn out the cookies onto a wire rack and allow them to cool.

Serving Suggestion: Serve with chocolate chip toppings.
Variation Tip: You can use natural peanut butter instead of the shake mixture.
Nutrition Per serving: Calories: 589; Fat: 34.6 g; Sat Fat: 11.5 g; Carbs: 64.4 g; Fiber: 0.1 g; Sugar: 53.5 g; Protein: 9.1 g.

299. Mint Cookies

Serving: 4
Difficulty: 1
Preparation Time: 10 minutes
Cooking Time: 15 minutes
Optavia Counts: 1 lean/ 0 green/ 1 healthy fat/ 0 condiments
Ingredients:

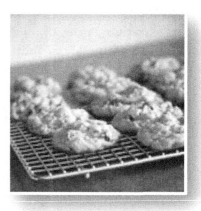

- 1 tbsp. liquid egg substitute
- 2 tbsp. unsweetened almond milk
- 2 Essential Chocolate Mint Cookie Crisp Bars
- 2 sachets Essential Decadent Double Chocolate Brownies

Directions:

1. Preheat the oven to 350°F. Line a cookie sheet with parchment paper.
2. Place the cookie bars in a food processor and pulse until fully crushed.
3. Transfer the crushed bars to a bowl with the other ingredients and mix until well blended.
4. Using a spoon, form 8 cookie dough balls from the mixture and place them onto the prepared cookie sheet. Press each ball slightly with your fingers.
5. Bake for 13 to 15 minutes.
6. Remove the cookie sheet from the oven and let it cool for 5 minutes on a wire rack.
7. Turn out the cookies onto the wire rack to cool before serving.

Serving Suggestion: These cookies are perfect as they are!
Variation Tip: Add some mint extract for an extra punch of flavor.
Nutrition Per serving: Calories: 175; Fat: 6.1 g; Sat Fat: 2.5 g; Carbs: 20.7 g; Fiber: 1.3 g; Sugar: 14.1 g; Protein: 9.8 g.

300. Parmesan Zucchini Rounds

Serving: 4
Difficulty: 1
Preparation Time: 25 minutes
Cooking Time: 20 minutes
Optavia Counts: 2 lean/ 2 green/ 1 healthy fat/ 2 condiments
Ingredients:

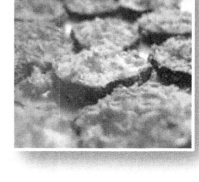

- 4 zucchinis; sliced
- 1 ½ cups Parmesan; grated
- ¼ cup parsley; chopped.
- 1 egg; whisked
- 1 egg white; whisked
- ½ tsp. garlic powder
- Cooking spray

Directions:

1. Take a bowl and mix the egg with egg whites, Parmesan, parsley, and garlic powder. Then whisk.
2. Dredge each zucchini slice in this mix, place them all in your Air Fryer's basket. Grease them with cooking spray and cook at 370°F for 20 minutes.
3. Divide between plates and serve as a side dish.

Nutrition: Calories: 183; Fat: 6 g; Fiber: 2 g; Carbs: 3 g; Protein: 8 g.

301. Green Bean Casserole

Serving: 4
Difficulty: 2
Preparation Time: 25 minutes
Cooking Time: 20 minutes
Optavia Counts: 1 lean/ 1 green/ 2 healthy fat/ 5 condiments
Ingredients:

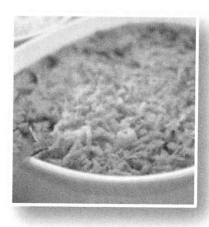

- 1 pound fresh green beans, edges trimmed
- ½ oz. pork rinds, finely ground
- 1 oz. full-fat cream cheese
- ½ cup heavy whipping cream.
- ¼ cup yellow onion, diced
- ½ cup white mushrooms, chopped
- ½ cup chicken broth
- 1 tbsp. unsalted butter
- ¼ tsp. xanthan gum

Directions:

1. Melt the butter in a preheated skillet.
2. Sauté the onion and mushrooms until soft and fragrant, for 3–5 minutes.
3. Add the heavy cream, cream cheese, and broth to the skillet. Lightly beat until smooth. Boil and then simmer. Put the xanthan gum in the pan and remove it from heat.
4. Cut green beans into 2-inch pieces and place in a 4-cup round pan. Pour sauce mixture over them and stir until covered. Fill the plate with ground pork rinds. Place in the fryer basket.
5. Set the temperature to 320°F and set the timer for 15 minutes. The top will be a golden and green bean fork when fully cooked. Serve hot.

Nutrition: Calories: 267; Protein: 3.6 g; Fat: 23.4 g; Carbs: 9.7 g.

BONUS RECIPES

302. Banana and Pumpkin Waffles

Serving: 4
Difficulty: 1
Preparation Time: 15 minutes
Cooking Time: 5 minutes
Optavia Counts: 1 lean/ 0 green/ 4 healthy fats/ 6 condiments
Ingredients:

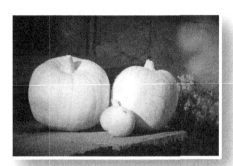

- 2 medium bananas
- 1 ½ tsp. ground cinnamon
- ½ cup coconut flour
- 2 tbsp. olive oil
- ½ tsp. ground cloves
- ¾ tsp. ground ginger
- 1 tsp. baking soda
- ½ tsp. ground nutmeg
- ½ cup almond flour
- 5 large eggs
- ¾ cup almond milk
- ½ cup pumpkin puree
- Salt

Directions:

1. Peel and slice the bananas. Preheat the waffle iron, and after that, grease it. In a big bowl, mix flour, baking soda, and spices. In a blender, put the remaining ingredients and pulse till smooth.
2. Add flour mixture and pulse till smooth. In preheated waffle iron, add the required quantity of mixture.
3. Cook approximately 4-5 minutes.
4. Repeat using the remaining mixture.

Nutrition: Calories: 357.2 kcal; Protein: 14 g; Fat: 28.5 g; Carbs: 19.7 g.

303. Chicken & Zucchini Pancakes

Serving: 4
Difficulty: 3
Preparation Time: 15 minutes
Cooking Time: 32 minutes
Optavia Counts: 2 lean/ 2 green/ 2 healthy fat/ 2 condiments
Ingredients:

- 4 cups zucchinis
- ¼ cup chicken
- ¼ cup scallion
- 1 egg
- ¼ cup coconut flour
- 1 tbsp. olive oil
- Salt
- Black pepper

Directions:

1. In a colander, place the shredded zucchini and sprinkle it with salt.
2. Set aside for about 8-10 minutes.
3. Squeeze the zucchinis well and transfer into a bowl.
4. Shred the chicken and finely chop the scallion.
5. In the bowl of zucchini, add the rest of the ingredients and mix until well combined.
6. In a large nonstick skillet, heat the oil over medium fire.
7. Add ¼ cup of zucchini mixture into the preheated skillet and spread in an even layer.

8. Cook for about 3-4 minutes per side.
9. Repeat with the remaining mixture.
10. Serve warm.

Nutrition: Calories: 89 kcal; Protein: 4.43 g; Fat: 6.87 g; Carbs: 2.68 g.

304. Damn Best Pork Chops

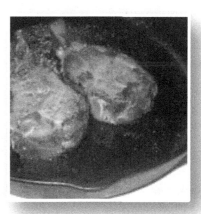

Serving: 2
Difficulty: 1
Preparation Time: 05 minutes
Cooking Time: 17 minutes
Optavia Counts: 1 lean/ 0 green/ 1 healthy fat/ 7 condiments
Ingredients:

- 2 pork chops - 1 ½ tsp. salt
- 2 tbsp. brown sugar
- 1 tbsp. paprika
- 1 ½ tsp. black pepper
- 2 tbsp. olive oil
- 1 tsp. ground mustard
- ½ tsp. onion powder
- ¼ tsp. garlic powder

Directions:

1. Preheat Air Fryer toaster oven to 400°F for 5 minutes. Wash pork chops with cool water and pat dry completely with a paper towel. In a bowl, add all the dry ingredients. Coat the pork chops with olive oil and brush in the mix. Brush it in well and liberally. Use all of the brushed mix for the 2 pork chops. Cook pork chops in Air Fryer toaster oven at 400°F for 12 minutes, turning pork chops over after 6 minutes if needed.

Nutrition: Calories: 198; Fat: 6 g; Protein: 25 g; Carbs: 10 g; Fiber: 0 g.

305. Mixed Vegetable Soup

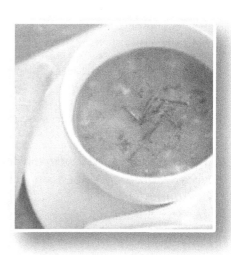

Serving: 4
Difficulty: 3
Preparation Time: 5 minutes
Cooking Time: 30 minutes
Optavia Counts: 0 lean/ 8 green/ 1 healthy fat/ 3 condiments
Ingredients:

- 1 tbsp. olive oil
- 1 chopped leek
- 1 chopped bok choy
- 2 chopped carrots
- 2 cloves minced garlic
- 1 chopped zucchini
- 1 chopped tomatoes
- 1 cup garbanzo beans
- 1 chopped potatoes
- 2 cups broth
- 1 tsp. basil
- ½ cup amaranth

Directions:

1. Sauté first four ingredients, add garlic for the last minute.
2. Add the rest of the ingredients and simmer on the stove for 25 minutes.

Nutrition: Calories: 241; Fat: 2 g; Fiber: 16 g; Carbs: 9 g; Protein: 22 g.

306. Air-Fried Bananas

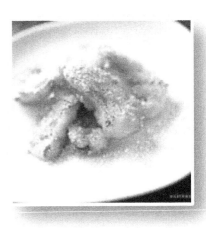

Serving: 4
Difficulty: 1
Preparation Time: 5 minutes
Cooking Time: 10 minutes
Optavia Counts: 1 lean/ 0 green/ 2 healthy fat/ 1 condiments
Ingredients:

- 1 tbsps. butter
- 2 eggs
- 2 bananas
- ½ cup corn flour
- 1 tsp. cinnamon sugar
- 1 cup Skilletko

Directions:

1. Preheat a skillet with the butter over medium heat. Put the Skilletko, turn and cook for 4 minutes; then move to a container.
2. Spin each in flour, Skilletko, egg blend, assemble them in Air Fryer's basket, grime with cinnamon sugar and cook at 280°F for 10 minutes.
3. Serve immediately.

Nutrition: Calories: 337; Fat: 3 g; Carbs: 20 g; Protein: 4 g.

307. Golden Turmeric Fish

Servings: 4
Difficulty: 1
Preparation Time: 20 minutes
Cooking Time: 30 minutes
Optavia Counts: 1 lean/ 1 green/ 1 healthy fat/ 8 condiments
Ingredients:

- 1 tbsp. unrefined coconut oil
- 1 tbsp. fresh lime juice
- 1 tbsp. grated fresh ginger
- 1 tsp. ground cilantro
- ½ tsp. ground turmeric
- ⅛ tsp. cayenne pepper
- 5-oz. red snapper fish fillets
- ½ tsp. salt - ¼ tsp. freshly ground black pepper
- Purchased mango chutney
- Chopped fresh cilantro

Directions:

1. In a shallow dish, blend the coconut oil, lime juice, ginger, cilantro, turmeric, and cayenne pepper together. I was using black pepper and salt to season the cod. Add a paste of coconut oil to the skinless sides of the cod. Place the fish in the broiler's greased pan. Broil for 10 minutes, or before fish flakes easily, at 4 inches. Serve with cilantro and chutney.

TIPS: Coconut oil is strong, much like shortening, and liquefies when it's humid. If you stir it into the spices to make the rub, it does not matter whether it is solid or liquid.

Nutrition: Calories: 268; Total fat: 9 g; Cholesterol: 52 mg; Sodium: 382 mg; Potassium: 630 mg; Carbs: 16 g; Fiber: 0 g; Sugar: 9 g; Protein: 29 g; Folate: 9 mc Calcium: 51 mg.

308. Squash Hash

Serving: 3
Difficulty: 1
Preparation Time: 2 minutes
Cooking Time: 10 minutes
Optavia Counts: 0 lean/ 0 green/ 0 healthy fat/ 4 condiments
Ingredients:

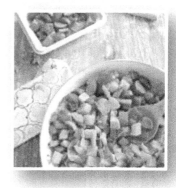

- 1 tsp. onion powder
- ½ cup finely chopped onion
- 2 cups spaghetti squash
- ½ tsp. sea salt

Directions:

1. Using paper towels, squeeze extra moisture from spaghetti squash.
2. Place the squash into a bowl; then add the salt, onion, and onion powder. Stir properly to mix them.
3. Coat a non-stick cooking skillet with cooking spray and place it over moderate heat. Add the spaghetti squash to the pan and cook for about 5 minutes.
4. Flip the hash browns using a spatula. Cook for 5 minutes until the desired crispness is reached. Serve.

Nutrition: Calories: 44; Fat: 0.6 g; Carbs: 9.7 g; Protein: 0.9 g.

309. Chicken & Veggie Quiche

Servings: 4
Difficulty: 2
Preparation Time: 15 minutes
Cooking Time: 20 minutes
Optavia Counts: 2 lean/ 7 green/ 1 healthy fat/ 1 condiments
Ingredients:

- 5 eggs
- ½ cup unsweetened almond milk
- Freshly ground black pepper, as required
- 1 cup cooked chicken, chopped
- ½ cup fresh baby spinach, chopped
- ½ cup fresh baby kale, chopped
- ¼ cup fresh mushrooms, sliced
- ¼ cup green bell pepper, seeded and chopped
- 1 scallion, chopped
- ¼ cup fresh cilantro, chopped
- 1 tbsp. fresh chives, minced

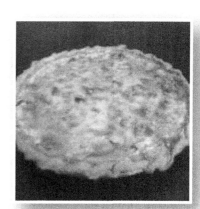

Directions:

1. Preheat your oven to 400°F. Lightly grease a pie dish.
2. In a large bowl, add the eggs, almond milk, salt and black pepper and beat well. Set aside.
3. In another bowl, add the chicken, vegetables, scallion and herbs. Mix well.
4. Place the chicken mixture in the bottom of the prepared pie dish.
5. Place the egg mixture over the chicken mixture evenly.
6. Bake for approximately 20 minutes or until a toothpick inserted in the center comes out clean.
7. Remove from the oven and set aside to cool for about 5-10 minutes before slicing.
8. Cut into desired size wedges and serve.

Nutrition Per Serving: Calories: 162; Fat: 8.1 g; Carbs: 2.9 g; Fiber: 0.6 g; Sugar: 1.1 g; Protein: 19.3 g; Sodium: 145 mg.

310. Chipotle Pork Loin

Serving: 3
Difficulty: 5
Preparation Time: 15 minutes.
Cooking Time: 6 hours.
Optavia Counts: 1 lean/ 0 green/ 0 healthy fat/ 2 condiments
Ingredients:

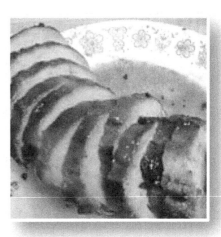

- 2 pounds boneless pork loin
- 1 tbsp. Garlic and Spring Onion Seasoning
- 1 tbsp. Cinnamon Chipotle Seasoning
- ¼ cup water

Directions:

1. Add pork loin, water, seasoning and chipotle to a slow cooker.
2. Cover and cook for 6 hours on low heat.
3. Serve warm.

Serving Suggestion: Serve the pork loin with sautéed carrots on the side.
Variation Tip: Drizzle parmesan cheese on top before serving.
Nutrition Per Serving: Calories: 345; Fat: 36 g; Sodium: 272mg; Carbs: 41 g; Fiber: 0.2 g; Sugar: 0.1 g; Protein: 22.5 g.

311. Chicken with Yellow Squash

Servings: 1
Difficulty: 1
Preparation Time: 15 minutes
Cooking Time: 17 minutes
Optavia Counts: 1 lean/ 1 green/ 1 healthy fat/ 5 condiments
Ingredients:

- 1 tbsp. olive oil, divided
- 1 ½ pounds skinless, boneless chicken breasts, cut into bite-sized pieces
- Salt and ground black pepper, as required
- 2 garlic cloves, minced
- 1 ½ pounds yellow squash, sliced
- 1 tbsp. fresh lemon juice
- 1 tsp. fresh lemon zest, grated finely
- 1 tbsp. fresh parsley, minced

Directions:

1. In a large wok, heat 1 tablespoon of oil over medium heat and stir fry chicken for about 6-8 minutes or until golden brown from all sides.
2. Transfer the chicken onto a plate.
3. In the same wok, heat the remaining oil over medium heat and sauté garlic for about 1 minute.
4. Add the squash slices and cook for about 5-6 minutes.
5. Stir in the chicken and cook for about 2 minutes.
6. Stir in the lemon juice, zest and parsley and remove from heat.
7. Serve hot.

Nutrition Per Serving: Calories: 203; Fat: 9 g; Carbs: 4.4 g; Fiber: 1.4 g; Sugar: 2.1 g; Protein: 26.8 g; Sodium: 81 mg.

312. Jalapeno Grilled Salmon with Tomato Confit

Servings: 1
Difficulty: 1
Preparation Time: 30 minutes
Cooking Time: 20 minutes
Optavia Counts: 1 lean/ 2 green/ 2 healthy fat/ 3 condiments
Ingredients:

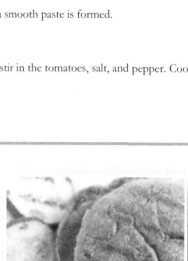

- 2 lb. salmon fillets
- 1 jalapeno
- 1 medium garlic cloves
- 1 tbsp. tomato paste
- 2 tbsp. olive oil
- Salt and pepper to taste
- 2 pints cherry tomatoes, halved
- 1 shallot, chopped

Directions:

1. Combine the jalapeno, garlic, tomato paste, and 2 tablespoons of oil in a mortar. Mix well until a smooth paste is formed.
2. Spread the spicy paste over the salmon and season it with salt and pepper.
3. Heat a grill pan over medium flame, then place the fish on the grill.
4. Cook on each side for 5–6 minutes.
5. For the confit, heat 1 tablespoon of oil in a skillet. Add the shallot and cook for 1 minute, then stir in the tomatoes, salt, and pepper. Cook for 2 minutes on high heat.
6. Serve the grilled salmon with the tomatoes.

Nutrition: Calories: 237; Fat: 14.5 g; Protein: 24 g; Carbohydrate: 4.4 g.

313. Zucchini Lean Pork Burger

Serving: 4
Difficulty: 2
Preparation Time: 20 minutes
Cooking Time: 25 minutes
Optavia Counts: 1 lean/ 1 green/ 1 healthy fat/ 4 condiments
Ingredients:

- 6 oz. zucchini
- Oil spray
- ¼ cup breadcrumbs
- 1 clove garlic
- 1 tbsp. red onion
- 1 pound lean pork
- 1 tsp. kosher salt, pepper

Directions:

1. Squeeze all the moisture very well from the zucchini with paper towels. In a bowl, mix the ground pork, zucchini, breadcrumbs, garlic, onion, salt, and pepper. Create 5 equal patties, 4 oz. each, ½ inch thick. Preheat the Air Fryer toaster oven to 370F. Now cook in a single layer in two batches for 10 minutes or cook until browned and cooked through from the center.

Nutrition: Calories: 212; Fat: 14 g; Protein: 15 g; Carbs: 5 g.

314. Mini Zucchini Bites

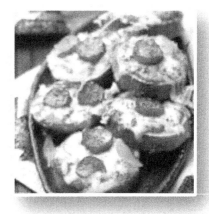

Serving: 3
Difficulty: 1
Preparation Time: 10 minutes
Cooking Time: 10 minutes
Optavia Counts: 0 lean/ 3 green/ 1 healthy fat/ 1 condiments
Ingredients:

- 2 medium sized Zucchini, cut into thick circles (2 greens)
- ½ pint Cherry tomatoes, halved (6 greens)
- ½ cup parmesan cheese, grated (1 healthy fat)
- Salt and pepper to taste (1 condiment)
- 1 tsp. chives, chopped (1 green)

Directions:

1. Preheat the oven to 390°F.
2. Add wax paper to a baking sheet.
3. Arrange the zucchini pieces.
4. Add the cherry halves to each zucchini slice.
5. Add parmesan cheese, chives, and sprinkle with salt and pepper.
6. Bake for 10 minutes. Serve.

Nutrition: Fat: 1 g; Protein: 7.3 g; Calories: 361.

315. Baked Chicken & Bell Peppers

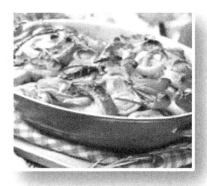

Servings: 2
Difficulty: 2
Preparation Time: 15 minutes
Cooking Time: 25 minutes
Optavia Counts: 1 lean/ 2 green/ 1 healthy fat/ 6 condiments
Ingredients:

- 1 pound boneless, skinless chicken breasts, cut into thin strips
- ½ of green bell pepper, seeded and cut into strips
- ½ of red bell pepper, seeded and cut into strips
- 1 medium onion, sliced
- 1 tbsp. olive oil
- ½ tsp. dried oregano
- 1 tsp. chili powder
- 1 ½ tsp. ground cumin
- 1 tsp. garlic powder
- Salt, as required

Directions:

1. Preheat your oven to 400°F.
2. In a bowl, add all the ingredients and mix well.
3. Place the chicken mixture into a 9x13-inch baking dish and spread in an even layer.
4. Bake for approximately 20-25 minutes or until chicken is done completely.
5. Serve hot.

Nutrition Per Serving: Calories: 314; Fat: 16.4 g; Carbs: 7 g; Fiber: 1.9 g; Sugar: 3 g; Protein: 34.1 g; Sodium: 156 mg.

MEAL PLAN 5&1

	Week 1	Week 2
Monday	297. Chicken Nuggets	290. Flavorsome Waffles
	300. Parmesan Zucchini Rounds	289. Cabbage and Radishes Mix
	277. Berry Mojito	296. Chocolate Donuts
	287. Brownie Cookies	277. Berry Mojito
	293. Delicious French Toast Sticks	288. Zucchini Spaghetti
	90. Tuna Salad (L&G)	129. Grilled Split Lobster (L&G)
Tuesday	280. Maple Pancakes	281. Brownie Pudding Cups
	286. Little Fudge Balls	298. Peanut Butter Cookies
	296. Chocolate Donuts	280. Maple Pancakes
	285. Mocha Cake	301. Green Bean Casserole
	279. Vanilla Shake	295. Pumpkin Waffles
	47. Bacon Frittata with Asparagus(L&G)	198. Creamy Pork Belly Rolls (L&G)
Wednesday	291. Richly Tasty Crepe	294. Shamrock Shake
	284. Tropical Smoothie Bowl	279. Vanilla Shake
	289. Cabbage and Radishes Mix	282. Tiramisu Shake
	294. Shamrock Shake	286. Little Fudge Balls
	290. Flavorsome Waffles	284. Tropical Smoothie Bowl
	33. Pasta with Avocado and Cream (L&G)	151. Chicken and Bok Choy (L&G)
Thursday	301. Green Bean Casserole	278. Vanilla Frappé
	298. Peanut Butter Cookies	300. Parmesan Zucchini Rounds
	295. Pumpkin Waffles	293. Delicious French Toast Sticks
	278. Vanilla Frappé	291. Richly Tasty Crepe
	282. Tiramisu Shake	299. Mint Cookies
	98. Beef with Mushrooms (L&G)	37. Meatball Lasagna (L&G)
	299. Mint Cookies	285. Mocha Cake
	288. Zucchini Spaghetti	297. Chicken Nuggets

Friday	281. Brownie Pudding Cups	287. Brownie Cookies
	292. Crunchy Cookies	292. Crunchy Cookies
	283. Potato Bagels	283. Potato Bagels
	153. Orange Chicken (L&G)	122. Pumpkin Smoothie (L&G)
Saturday	301. Green Bean Casserole	283. Potato Bagels
	285. Mocha Cake	279. Vanilla Shake
	288. Zucchini Spaghetti	277. Berry Mojito
	279. Vanilla Shake	280. Maple Pancakes
	281. Brownie Pudding Cups	285. Mocha Cake
	166. Quinoa Porridge (L&G)	125. Grilled Salmon with Cucumber Dill Sauce (L&G)
Sunday	289. Cabbage and Radishes Mix	300. Parmesan Zucchini Rounds
	295. Pumpkin Waffles	278. Vanilla Frappé
	294. Shamrock Shake	286. Little Fudge Balls
	280. Maple Pancakes	289. Cabbage and Radishes Mix
	298. Peanut Butter Cookies	291. Richly Tasty Crepe
	148. Vinegar Chicken (L&G)	227. Risotto with Green Beans and Sweet Potatoes (L&G)

	Week 3	Week 4
Monday	298. Peanut Butter Cookies	298. Peanut Butter Cookies
	295. Pumpkin Waffles	287. Brownie Cookies
	284. Tropical Smoothie Bowl	279. Vanilla Shake
	281. Brownie Pudding Cups	284. Tropical Smoothie Bowl
	287. Brownie Cookies	294. Shamrock Shake
	34. Spaghetti Squash with Cheese and Pesto (L&G)	251. Chicken Enchilada Soup (L&G)
Tuesday	290. Flavorsome Waffles	292. Crunchy Cookies
	292. Crunchy Cookies	296. Chocolate Donuts
	282. Tiramisu Shake	285. Mocha Cake
	301. Green Bean Casserole	290. Flavorsome Waffles
	294. Shamrock Shake	289. Cabbage and Radishes Mix
	97. Veggies and Fish Bake (L&G)	46. Tuna Cobbler (L&G)

Wednesday	296. Chocolate Donuts	297. Chicken Nuggets
	297. Chicken Nuggets	288. Zucchini Spaghetti
	288. Zucchini Spaghetti	291. Richly Tasty Crepe
	299. Mint Cookies	281. Brownie Pudding Cups
	293. Delicious French Toast Sticks	283. Potato Bagels
	119. Plum and Avocado Smoothie (L&G)	140. Tilapia Tacos (L&G)
Thursday	281. Brownie Pudding Cups	299. Mint Cookies
	295. Pumpkin Waffles	280. Maple Pancakes
	294. Shamrock Shake	278. Vanilla Frappé
	287. Brownie Cookies	301. Green Bean Casserole
	284. Tropical Smoothie Bowl	295. Pumpkin Waffles
	294. Air Fryer Pork Chop & Broccoli (L&G)	206. Roasted Pepper Pork Prosciutto (L&G)
Friday	298. Peanut Butter Cookies	300. Parmesan Zucchini Rounds
	283. Potato Bagels	282. Tiramisu Shake
	301. Green Bean Casserole	286. Little Fudge Balls
	279. Vanilla Shake	277. Berry Mojito
	293. Delicious French Toast Sticks	293. Delicious French Toast Sticks
	210. Zucchini Omelet (L&G)	225. Beef with Broccoli or Cauliflower Rice (L&G)
Saturday	297. Chicken Nuggets	288. Zucchini Spaghetti
	288. Zucchini Spaghetti	281. Brownie Pudding Cups
	290. Flavorsome Waffles	278. Vanilla Frappé
	282. Tiramisu Shake	292. Crunchy Cookies
	296. Chocolate Donuts	283. Potato Bagels
	100. Green Apple Smoothie (L&G)	86. Turkey Meatballs with Herbs (L&G)
Sunday	280. Maple Pancakes	280. Maple Pancakes
	285. Mocha Cake	293. Delicious French Toast Sticks
	286. Little Fudge Balls	301. Green Bean Casserole

278. Vanilla Frappé

285. Mocha Cake

289. Cabbage and Radishes Mix

294. Shamrock Shake

37. Meatball Lasagna (L&G)

25. Salmon Burgers (L&G)

MEAL PLAN 4&2&1

	Week 1	Week 2
Monday	287. Brownie Cookies	289. Cabbage and Radishes Mix
	292. Crunchy Cookies	285. Mocha Cake
	278. Vanilla Frappé	282. Tiramisu Shake
	283. Potato Bagels	301. Green Bean Casserole
	29. Chicken Omelet (L&G)	140. Tilapia Tacos (L&G)
	104. Green Mango Smoothie (L&G)	163. Chicken & Zucchini Muffins (L&G)
	70. Taco Stuffed Portobellos (Snack)	53. Mint Chocolate Cheesecake Muffins (Snack)
Tuesday	291. Richly Tasty Crepe	278. Vanilla Frappé
	299. Mint Cookies	293. Delicious French Toast Sticks
	294. Shamrock Shake	283. Potato Bagels
	297. Chicken Nuggets	288. Zucchini Spaghetti
	28. Zucchini Frittata (L&G)	172. Baked Cheesy Eggplant with Marinara (L&G)
	152. Chicken & Strawberry Lettuce Wraps (L&G)	191. Mozzarella Pork Belly Cheese (L&G)
	71. Mini Pepper Nachos (Snack)	59. Personal Biscuit Pizza (Snack)
Wednesday	282. Tiramisu Shake	277. Berry Mojito
	285. Mocha Cake	298. Peanut Butter Cookies
	295. Pumpkin Waffles	296. Chocolate Donuts
	290. Flavorsome Waffles	284. Tropical Smoothie Bowl
	36. Fish Lettuce Tacos (L&G)	180. Green Pea Guacamole (L&G)
	232. Cheesy Cauliflower Soup (L&G)	121. Lean and Green Smoothie 1 (L&G)
	67. Pinto's & Cheese Fueling Hack (Snack)	49. Cauliflower Pizza with Chicken & Tzatziki (Snack)

Thursday	284. Tropical Smoothie Bowl	291. Richly Tasty Crepe
	298. Peanut Butter Cookies	297. Chicken Nuggets
	279. Vanilla Shake	292. Crunchy Cookies
	277. Berry Mojito	295. Pumpkin Waffles
	182. Coconut Pancakes (L&G)	303. Chicken & Zucchini Pancakes (L&G)
	80. Winter Salad (L&G)	190. Pork Dumplings with Sauce (L&G)
	69. Grilled Mahi with Jicama Slaw (Snack)	54. Neapolitan Froyo Popsicles (Snack)
Friday	289. Cabbage and Radishes Mix	290. Flavorsome Waffles
	288. Zucchini Spaghetti	300. Parmesan Zucchini Rounds
	293. Delicious French Toast Sticks	287. Brownie Cookies
	300. Parmesan Zucchini Rounds	279. Vanilla Shake
	30. Chicken Pesto Pasta (L&G)	160. Basil Duck Fillet (L&G)
	88. Pan Fried Salmon (L&G)	210. Zucchini Omelet (L&G)
	64. Buffalo Cauliflower Wings (Snack)	66. Very Veggie Dip (Snack)
Saturday	296. Chocolate Donuts	299. Mint Cookies
	301. Green Bean Casserole	294. Shamrock Shake
	291. Richly Tasty Crepe	289. Cabbage and Radishes Mix
	299. Mint Cookies	285. Mocha Cake
	31. Crab Cakes (L&G)	220. Plant-Powered Pancakes (L&G)
	228. Maple Lemon Tempeh Cubes (L&G)	204. Crispy Pork Cutlets (L&G)
	72. Curried Chicken Salad Wraps (Snack)	73. Cilantro Lime Fish (Snack)
Sunday	287. Brownie Cookies	301. Green Bean Casserole
	292. Crunchy Cookies	278. Vanilla Frappé
	278. Vanilla Frappé	293. Delicious French Toast Sticks
	283. Potato Bagels	283. Potato Bagels
	42. Chicken Cordon Bleu (L&G)	189. Pork Chop with Brussels Sprout (L&G)
	77. Cheesy Zucchini (L&G)	218. Carrot Cake Oatmeal (L&G)

61. Caprese Pizza Bites (Snack)	70. Taco Stuffed Portobellos (Snack)

	Week 3	Week 4
Monday	297. Chicken Nuggets	279. Vanilla Shake
	299. Mint Cookies	298. Peanut Butter Cookies
	290. Flavorsome Waffles	285. Mocha Cake
	279. Vanilla Shake	290. Flavorsome Waffles
	228. Maple Lemon Tempeh Cubes (L&G)	27. Mini Mac in a Bowl (L&G)
	81. Energizing Mocha Smoothie (L&G)	227. Risotto with Green Beans and Sweet Potatoes (L&G)
	51. Thin Mint Cookies (Snack)	63. Smash Potato Grilled Cheese (Snack)
Tuesday	295. Pumpkin Waffles	293. Delicious French Toast Sticks
	283. Potato Bagels	278. Vanilla Frappé
	278. Vanilla Frappé	301. Green Bean Casserole
	296. Chocolate Donuts	295. Pumpkin Waffles
	41. Avocados Stuffed with Salmon (L&G)	95. Salmon with Pineapple (L&G)
	156. Chicken & Broccoli Bake (L&G)	206. Roasted Pepper Pork Prosciutto (L&G)
	50. 2-Ingredient Peanut Butter Energy Bites (Snack)	58. Skinny Chicken Queso (Snack)
Wednesday	300. Parmesan Zucchini Rounds	291. Richly Tasty Crepe
	277. Berry Mojito	288. Zucchini Spaghetti
	282. Tiramisu Shake	289. Cabbage and Radishes Mix
	284. Tropical Smoothie Bowl	297. Chicken Nuggets
	48. Spaghetti Squash Casserole (L&G)	127. Basil 'n Lime-Chili Clams (L&G)
	78. Veggie Crusty Pizza (L&G)	177. Baked Potato Topped with Cream Cheese and Olives (L&G)
	63. Smash Potato Grilled Cheese (Snack)	65. Cheddar & Chive Savory Smashed

Day		
		Potato Waffles (Snack)
Thursday	292. Crunchy Cookies	283. Potato Bagels
	287. Brownie Cookies	277. Berry Mojito
	293. Delicious French Toast Sticks	294. Shamrock Shake
	288. Zucchini Spaghetti	282. Tiramisu Shake
	34. Spaghetti Squash with Cheese and Pesto (L&G)	125. Grilled Salmon with Cucumber Dill Sauce (L&G)
	235. Corner-Filling Soup (L&G)	84. Free Tofu (L&G)
	57. Mini Peanut Butter Cups (Snack)	51. Thin Mint Cookies (Snack)
Friday	298. Peanut Butter Cookies	292. Crunchy Cookies
	294. Shamrock Shake	284. Tropical Smoothie Bowl
	301. Green Bean Casserole	287. Brownie Cookies
	285. Mocha Cake	296. Chocolate Donuts
	162. Chicken & Asparagus Frittata (L&G)	46. Tuna Cobbler (L&G)
	229. Quinoa with Vegetables (L&G)	163. Chicken & Zucchini Muffins (L&G)
	56. Cranberry Sweet Potato Muffins (Snack)	60. Mini Cranberry Orange Spiced Cheesecake (Snack)
Saturday	289. Cabbage and Radishes Mix	300. Parmesan Zucchini Rounds
	291. Richly Tasty Crepe	299. Mint Cookies
	290. Flavorsome Waffles	278. Vanilla Frappé
	282. Tiramisu Shake	292. Crunchy Cookies
	33. Pasta with Avocado and Cream (L&G)	239. Curried Pumpkin Soup (L&G)
	82. Flavored Sandwich Filling (L&G)	164. Chicken & Bell Pepper Muffins (L&G)
	70. Personal Portobello Mushroom Pizzas (Snack)	72. Curried Chicken Salad Wraps (Snack)
Sunday	280. Maple Pancakes	285. Mocha Cake
	285. Mocha Cake	290. Flavorsome Waffles
	286. Little Fudge Balls	293. Delicious French Toast Sticks
	278. Vanilla Frappé	278. Vanilla Frappé

44. Lemon Parmesan Salmon (L&G)	38. Lettuce Salad with Beef Strips (L&G)
111. Watermelon Strawberry Smoothie (L&G)	117. Watermelon Kale Smoothie (L&G)
61. Caprese Pizza Bites (Snack)	70. Taco Stuffed Portobellos (Snack)

CONCLUSION

Numerous studies have shown that lean and green diets prevent not only cardiovascular diseases but also mental disorders. As a result, a plant-based diet is ideal for anyone seeking to live a healthy lifestyle while lowering their risk of illness. Consequently, it's essential to eat healthy plant-based food to live longer and be more beneficial.

A lean and green diet is much more than just a way to reduce the number of animal products in your diet. There are many advantages of following this regimen, one of which is the fact that it is very inexpensive. It not only requires eating unprocessed, nutrient-dense foods, but it also implies that you are less likely to become unwell as a result of toxins contained in meat and dairy products. This type of food usually takes longer to eat, leaving less room for other food on your plate and can leave you feeling hungry sooner than if you had eaten something typical like hamburgers or hot dogs. However, it's important to note that all meals should be nutritious and accompanied by healthy ingredients. It's also vital to learn about the right types of lean and green food so there are no deficiencies.

Green juices are trendy nowadays. Many people have started drinking green juices prepared with nutritious ingredients. They are very healthy and can be made at home with vegetables that you probably have in your refrigerator. Fresh fruits and vegetables can be juiced, but it is also possible to use leafy greens, cucumber, apple, lemon, and watercress for vegan green juice recipes. To make your green juice more filling, you can add wheatgrass or spirulina powder to it. You can drink green juices either on their own or as a complement to a meal.

Many people believe that eating lean and green is a difficult lifestyle because they think they must forego so many delicious foods and ingredients. However, after reading this book, you will know how to cook delicious vegan food that will bring you all the benefits of this lifestyle. You don't have to give up your favorite dishes; you can still eat burgers, meatballs, and grilled chicken. Just make sure these are made with healthy ingredients, so you are eating nutritious food. Make sure to have a variety of foods, so there are vitamins and minerals in your diet. You can include fresh fruits, green juices, and other healthy meals in your diet, but you must get enough protein in your body by eating soy products or other types of beans. There are many delicious recipes for sweets that have the same texture or taste as traditional desserts made with eggs or milk. If you want to be healthier and live longer, you should know that meals prepared with animal products are not as nutritious as meals made with plant-based foods.

Made in the USA
Middletown, DE
20 March 2022